Brief Dynamic and Interpersonal Therapy

Second Edition

CONCISE
GUIDES

Robert E. Hales, M.D.
Series Editor

CONCISE GUIDE TO
Brief Dynamic and Interpersonal Therapy

Second Edition

Hanna Levenson, Ph.D.

Stephen F. Butler, Ph.D.

Theodore A. Powers, Ph.D.

Bernard D. Beitman, M.D.

American Psychiatric Publishing, Inc.

Washington, DC
London, England

Manufactured in the United States of America on acid-free paper
06 05 04 03 02   5 4 3 2 1
Second Edition

Typeset in Adobe's Times and Helvetica

American Psychiatric Publishing, Inc.
1400 K Street, N.W.
Washington, DC 20005
www.appi.org

Library of Congress Cataloging-in-Publication Data
Concise guide to brief dynamic and interpersonal therapy / Hanna Levenson ... [et al.].—
2nd ed.
        p. cm.
    Previously ed cataloged according to rules under Levenson.
Includes bibliographical references and index.
ISBN 1-58562-048-3 (alk. paper)
    1. Psychodynamic psychotherapy. 2. Brief psychotherapy. I. Levenson, Hanna, 1945-

    RC489.P72 L48 2002
616.89′14—dc21

                                                                                    2002022566

British Library Cataloguing in Publication Data
A CIP record is available from the British Library.

CONTENTS

LIST OF TABLES

5 Time-Limited Dynamic Psychotherapy

6 Short-Term Dynamic Therapy for Patients With Posttraumatic Stress Disorder

7 Brief Dynamic Psychotherapy for Patients With Substance Abuse Disorders

8 Time-Limited Group Therapy

9 The Reciprocal Relationship Between Pharmacotherapy and Psychotherapy

LIST OF FIGURES

ABOUT THE AUTHORS

Hanna Levenson, Ph.D., is the Founder of the Levenson Institute for Training (LIFT) and Director of the Brief Psychotherapy Program at California Pacific Medical Center in San Francisco. She also maintains a private practice in San Francisco and Oakland, California. For 20 years she was Clinical Professor in the Department of Psychiatry at the University of California School of Medicine. Past positions include Director of Brief Therapy Training at the Veterans Administration Medical Centers in San Francisco and Palo Alto, California.

Stephen F. Butler, Ph.D., is Senior Vice President and Chief Science Officer at Inflexxion (formerly Innovative Training Systems), a research and consulting firm based in Massachusetts that develops scientifically based solutions in the areas of health education, prevention, and disease management. Before serving in this position, he held faculty appointments in the Vanderbilt University Psychology Department and the Psychiatry Department of the Medical College of Virginia. He was also Director of Psychology at Nashua Brookside Hospital, Nashua, New Hampshire.

Theodore A. Powers, Ph.D., is an Assistant Professor in the Department of Psychology at the University of Massachusetts Dartmouth. Previously, he was Clinical Director of the Short-Term Therapies Unit at Massachusetts General Hospital and an Instructor at Harvard Medical School.

Bernard D. Beitman, M.D., is Professor and Chairman in the Department of Psychiatry and Neurology at the University of Missouri–Columbia School of Medicine.

INTRODUCTION

to the Concise Guides Series

The Concise Guides Series from American Psychiatric Publishing, Inc., provides, in an accessible format, practical information for psychiatrists, psychiatry residents, and medical students working in a variety of treatment settings, such as inpatient psychiatry units, outpatient clinics, consultation-liaison services, and private office settings. The Concise Guides are meant to complement the more detailed information to be found in lengthier psychiatry texts.

The Concise Guides address topics of special concern to psychiatrists in clinical practice. The books in this series contain a detailed table of contents, along with an index, tables, figures, and other charts for easy access. The books are designed to fit into a lab coat pocket or jacket pocket, which makes them a convenient source of information. References have been limited to those most relevant to the material presented.

Robert E. Hales, M.D., M.B.A.
Series Editor, Concise Guides

INTRODUCTION

■ FOCUS OF THE BOOK

Psychodynamic Orientation

In writing this book, we have taken the position that the clinician who is trying to institute time-limited or time-efficient approaches needs to operate from a systematic, theoretically based model. As Kurt Lewin, a social psychologist, is credited with stating, "There is nothing so practical as a good theory" (Marrow 1969, p. viii). We have chosen to focus on psychodynamically based or dynamically informed models, but not because psychodynamic theory is the be-all and end-all of all approaches. In fact, there is now ample empirical evidence that most schools of therapy achieve approximately the same magnitude of outcomes, and all do better than no treatment or various types of control groups (Olinsky and Howard 1995).

We have instead selected various psychodynamic treatment models to present here because "dynamic psychiatry simply provides a coherent conceptual framework within which all treatments are prescribed. Regardless of whether the treatment is dynamic psychotherapy or pharmacotherapy, it is dynamically informed" (Gabbard 2000,

Portions of this chapter were reprinted from Levenson H, Hales RE: "Brief Psychodynamically Informed Therapy for Medically Ill Patients," in *Medical-Psychiatric Practice,* 1st Edition, Vol. 2. Edited by Stoudemire A, Fogel BS. Washington, DC, American Psychiatric Press, 1993, pp. 3–37. Copyright 1993, American Psychiatric Press. Used with permission.

p. 4). This viewpoint is supported by the conclusion of the joint task force of the Association for Academic Psychiatry and the American Association of Directors of Psychiatry Residency Training (Mohl et al. 1990), which held that psychodynamic psychotherapy is critical in general psychiatry education. In short, "a deep, usable understanding of and ability to apply clinically the concepts of a dynamic unconscious, transference and countertransference, and mental defense mechanisms are central to being an effective pharmacotherapist, behavior therapist, inpatient psychiatrist, consultation psychiatrist, and, perhaps, even a laboratory research psychiatrist" (p. 9).

A recent national random survey of 4,000 mental health professionals (Davidovitz and Levenson 1995; Levenson and Davidovitz 2000) found that one-half of psychiatrists and one-quarter of psychologists and social workers identified themselves as having a purely psychodynamic orientation. An additional 40% overall held an eclectic or integrative stance. Thus the psychodynamic perspective has been and remains quite robust and fundamental to the day-to-day practice of clinicians.

Throughout this book, we define *psychodynamically informed therapies* as those that consider, to a greater or lesser degree, the importance of early development, unconscious determinants of behavior, conflict, the therapeutic relationship between therapist and patient (including transference and countertransference), patients' resistance to the work, and repetitive behavior. We do not, however, present psychodynamic models that use complex, highly inferential constructs (e.g., oral, anal, and phallic stages of development) or that require the adoption of an elaborate, metapsychological framework with unclear behavioral referents (e.g., id, ego, and superego). Rather, we have selected dynamic approaches that adhere closely to the observable data, because they have been shown to be quite clinically useful and didactically teachable.

Interpersonal Focus

In the second edition of this book, we have chosen to make explicit the importance we place on an interpersonal perspective. Within psychoanalytic theory and practice, there has been a paradigm shift from a one-person to a two-person psychology. This shift is away from the Freudian position of viewing the biological discharge of drives as determining the development of personality and toward recognizing innate motivations to maintain interpersonal relatedness. In fact, Harry Stack Sullivan (1953), one of the early proponents of interpersonal theory, defined personality as "that relatively enduring pattern of *recurrent interpersonal situations* which characterize the human life" (p. 111; emphasis added).

Accumulating empirical evidence (especially from research on child development) points to how human beings are fundamentally hardwired to seek attachment to others. Reciprocally, interpersonal relationships influence brain function. For example, Siegel (1999), citing neurobiological evidence, suggests that "relationships early in life may shape the very structures that create representations of experience and allow a coherent view of the world" (p. 4). In this way, interpersonal experiences directly influence the means by which we mentally construe reality. Messer and Warren (1995) point out that various scientific, cultural, social, and clinical factors account for the fact that most contemporary psychoanalytic schools are becoming less drive oriented and more relational. For the practicing clinician, this shift to a more interpersonal stance affects what gets defined as pathology, how one formulates the case, what interventions are considered most helpful, and how outcome is evaluated.

■ BRIEF PSYCHOTHERAPY

To the novice reader, it may seem that brief psychotherapy is a recent phenomenon brought on by the advent of managed care and third-party payers as a result of the shrinking mental health dollar. However, for years patients themselves have been electing to be treated briefly by choosing to stay in therapy for an average of six to eight sessions, regardless of the type of outpatient treatment they are receiving (Levenson and Burg 2000). These findings hold even for treatments that are intended to be long term (Pekarik and

Wierzbicki 1986). It has been estimated that 90% of all patients leave treatment by the tenth session. Although we do not know precisely the reasons for these dropouts, improvement data indicate that approximately 50% of patients report considerable benefit by the eighth session (Howard et al. 1986).

Most patients who present for therapy are in emotional pain. They want to have their pain alleviated as soon as possible. Most of them are not fascinated by their psyches, nor are they pursuing mental health perfection.

These consumer-defined brief therapies, or what have been called *naturally occurring brief therapies,* are quite different from therapies that are planned from the start to make the most of limited time. Brief therapies by default, which has been the norm, are in contrast to the therapies presented here, which are brief therapies by design.

Outcome data for planned short-term therapies indicate that the average patient receiving brief therapy does better than 80% of untreated control subjects (Koss and Shiang 1993). In fact, empirical studies have failed to demonstrate that long-term therapies achieve better measurable outcomes than do short-term. "Perhaps no other finding has been reported with greater regularity in the mental health literature than the equal clinical effect of time-limited and time-unlimited psychotherapy" (Bloom 2001, p. 76).

Today, because of limited mental health resources, emphasis on accountability, the concerns of third-party payers, and consumer need, there is an increasing demand for mental health professionals to use briefer therapeutic approaches. In the Davidovitz and Levenson (1995) national practitioner survey, 84% of all clinicians said that they are doing some form of planned brief therapy for a portion of their practices.

Brief Dynamic Approaches

Traditionally, 25 sessions has been defined as marking the upper limit of brief dynamic therapies (Levenson and Burg 2000), but in practice, the range may be a few as 1 (Bloom 1997) or as many as

40 (Sifneos 1987). Although many health maintenance organizations have a stated limit of 20 sessions per year, usually for crisis intervention or medical necessity, their average is closer to 6 sessions. Other settings impose various time limits, but most fall between 6 and 20 visits.

Recently, however, there has been a movement away from considering brief therapy merely in terms of the number of sessions. Instead, researchers, theoreticians, and clinicians are talking about time-attentive models that try to make every session count, regardless of the length of treatment. Here the emphasis is on the therapist's and the patient's time-limited attitudes, and terms such as *time-effective*, *time-sensitive*, and *cost-effective* seem more relevant.

As expected in the nationwide practitioner survey (Davidovitz and Levenson 1995), psychodynamically oriented therapists reported that they spent fewer hours in brief therapy than did their colleagues with other theoretical orientations. Because the dynamic therapists made up such a large proportion of the sample, however, they were responsible for one-fourth of all the brief therapy being conducted in the United States. Unfortunately, the survey data also indicate that the psychodynamic practitioners who were doing brief therapy had received significantly less training in it, felt less skilled to do it, and judged it to be less effective than did their colleagues trained in other orientations.

These findings are alarming from a consumer perspective. It is now widely accepted that brief therapy is not dehydrated long-term therapy (Cummings 1986) nor just less of the same (Peake et al. 1988), but rather requires specialized training in its own methodology (Levenson et al., in press). Therapists who are trained in brief therapy and follow specified methods have better outcomes than those who do not (Burlingame et al. 1989; O'Malley et al. 1988; Rounsaville et al. 1988), and trained clinicians feel that they are better skilled in brief therapy than are their untrained counterparts (Levenson et al. 1995). Yet it seems apparent that a major discrepancy exists between the demand and the supply of professionals who are prepared to use time-efficient methods effectively. This *Concise Guide* on brief dynamic and interpersonal therapies is a step in the direction of helping to educate both beginning and experienced clinicians in the strategies and techniques of these models.

Qualities That Define Brief Dynamic Therapy

In a content analysis of books and articles addressing the essential features that distinguish brief dynamic from long-term dynamic therapy, Levenson et al. (in press) found a number of fundamental qualities pertinent to brief therapy that were repeatedly mentioned. Table 1–1 contains a list of these qualities, rank ordered in terms of the frequency with which they are mentioned in the literature. This list provides a consensual, operational definition of short-term dynamic psychotherapy. All of the therapies presented in this book manifest these characteristics to some extent.

■ VALUES AND ATTITUDES

Unfortunately, it is not just for lack of didactic information that there are not more psychodynamically oriented therapists who feel more skilled in applying brief interventions. Because many dynamic clinicians operate from an orientation that has valued long-term, depth-oriented work, they have resistances toward learning short-term methods despite clinical advances and outcome data that demonstrate their effectiveness. Such clinicians may hold a number of myths or erroneous beliefs that make them reluctant to learn briefer interventions. Table 1–2 lists some sources of resistance toward briefer therapies and can be reviewed in order to assess one's own resistance level.

Budman and Gurman (1988) proposed that the value system of the long-term therapist is significantly different from that of the short-term therapist. They suggested that one of the critical criteria for defining the nature of brief therapy is "a state of mind of the therapist and of the patient" (p. 278), rather than the number of sessions or the length of treatment. These authors postulated eight dominant values pertaining to the ideal manner in which long-term therapy is practiced. They then contrasted these values with the cor-

TABLE 1–1.   **Qualities that define brief dynamic psychotherapy**

Limited focus and limited goals
Time limits and time management
Specific selection criteria
Therapist activity
Need to develop a therapeutic alliance quickly
Rapid assessment
Termination
Optimism on the part of the therapist
Treatment contract

Source. Levenson et al., in press.

TABLE 1–2.   **Sources of resistance against short-term dynamic psychotherapy**

1. The belief that more is better
2. Therapeutic perfectionism
3. Confusion of patient's interests with therapist's interests
4. Demands of greater activity and intense alertness
5. May be less profitable and dependable
6. Therapist's conflicts around separation and loss
7. Therapist's conflicts around attachment with new patients
8. Therapist's negative reaction to being told what to do
9. The need to be needed
10. Insecurities regarding one's own skill
11. Anxiety over the loss of one's professional role
12. Overconcern for "successful" termination

Source. Bauer and Kobos 1987; Hoyt 1985; Martin and Schurtman 1985.

responding ideal values that are pertinent to the practice of short-term therapy. Table 1–3 lists the comparative dominant values of the long-term and the short-term therapist.

In an empirical study, Bolter et al. (1990) found that for two of the eight dominant values, responses differed between therapists who prefer doing long-term therapy and those who prefer short-term approaches. Specifically, short-term therapists believed more strongly that psychological change occurs after therapy (value 4)

TABLE 1-3. Comparative dominant values of the long-term and the short-term therapist

	Long-term therapist	Short-term therapist
1.	Change in basic character	Least radical intervention, does not believe in the notion of cure.
2.	Significant psychological change is unlikely in everyday life.	Adult developmental perspective; psychological change is inevitable.
3.	Presenting problems reflect more basic pathology.	Presenting problems are taken seriously (although not always at face value).
4.	"Be there" as patient makes significant changes.	Many changes will occur after therapy.
5.	Therapy has a timeless quality; therapist practices patience.	Therapy is finite; therapist is active.
6.	Fiscal convenience of maintaining long-term patients.	Fiscal issues are muted by an organizational structure.
7.	Psychotherapy is almost always benign and useful.	Psychotherapy is sometimes useful, sometimes harmful.
8.	Therapy is the most important part of the patient's life.	Being in the world is more important than being in therapy.

Source. Adapted from Budman SH, Gurman AS: *Theory and Practice of Brief Psychotherapy.* New York, Guilford Press, 1988, p. 11. Copyright 1988, Guilford Press. Used with permission.

and that setting time limits intensifies the therapeutic work (value 5). However, the results also indicated that clinicians with a psychodynamic orientation (in contrast to those trained in cognitive-behavioral models) were more likely to believe that therapy is necessary for change (value 2), that therapy should be open ended (value 5), and that ambitious goals are desirable (value 1). Thus, these findings suggest that although one's preferred approach (short- versus long-term) is related to therapeutic values, the therapist's theoretical orientation (psychodynamic versus cognitive-behavioral) also plays a significant role.

In the national practitioner survey (Davidovitz and Levenson 1995), 90% of psychodynamic therapists said they preferred doing long-term and moderately long-term therapy. Thus, we can expect that a sizable number of therapists are in conflict—doing brief work that they do not believe in, feel skilled in, or prefer to do, but out of economic or administrative constraints feel pressured to do. For these reasons, dynamic therapists need training opportunities that focus not only on acquiring mastery of new brief therapy techniques, but also on encouraging the development of a different set of values and attitudes (Levenson and Strupp 1999).

We therefore hope that this *Concise Guide* will not only help educate clinicians that brief psychodynamic approaches have much to offer in the meaningful treatment of people presenting for help but will also foster more positive and optimistic attitudes toward the use of brief therapy.

■ SPECIFIC MODELS PRESENTED

Eight psychodynamic brief therapy models are presented in this volume:

1. Supportive therapy
2. Time-limited therapy
3. Interpersonal therapy
4. Time-limited dynamic psychotherapy
5. Short-term dynamic therapy for posttraumatic stress disorder

6. Brief dynamic therapy for substance abuse disorders
7. Time-limited group therapy
8. Pharmacotherapy and psychotherapy integration

These eight models were chosen because they represent well-established, short-term approaches to clinical issues that therapists commonly encounter in their clinical practices. In addition, most of them have clearly defined intervention techniques and formulation strategies that should help the novice as well as the experienced clinician who wishes to use brief interventions in a more informed manner. Many of the models exemplify an interpersonal perspective. In keeping with this focus, in this second edition we have added an entirely new chapter covering brief group therapy. We have also tried to select models that could be used within the 10- to 20-session time frame of most managed care settings. Nonetheless, many of these approaches are equally applicable regardless of the length of the treatment. (One notable exception is time-limited therapy, discussed in Chapter 3.)

The foregoing list is not meant to be exhaustive or representative. We do think, however, that the psychodynamically informed practitioner who is knowledgeable about these eight models has an enormous armamentarium of clinical interventions to help patients in a time-efficient and effective manner.

In seven of the chapters, a particular model is discussed in terms of its overall framework, selection criteria, goals, therapeutic tasks and strategies, empirical support, and relevance for managed care. Clinical cases are used to illustrate the application of each model. In the last chapter, a discussion of psychopharmacotherapy is provided from the standpoint of the dynamically informed use of medications.

At the beginning of each chapter are listed the various presenting problems we think are most suitable for treatment by that particular approach. Although psychodynamic models have often been used generically to treat all individuals for every problem, we are impressed with how each model seems more applicable to certain types of problems and/or to particular patients. By highlighting these relevant problems, we hope the practitioner will be guided to consider using a particular approach for reasons other than previous indoctrination, bias, or lack of knowledge.

Some problems are so prominent or overwhelming that the clinician should first consider using a treatment specifically designed to treat them. For example, for significant substance abuse, one should use models designed to treat that problem before considering treatment for other (presumably less pressing) problems. The sophisticated and experienced clinician will be able to combine aspects from various approaches to treat more precisely any combination of presenting problems. Because all of these approaches are basically psychodynamic in orientation, they can maintain an overall coherence if several are blended. The eight treatment models can be characterized by the degree to which they use supportive versus expressive techniques, focus on acute versus chronic problems, and target changes in symptoms versus personality.

Because this a concise guide, the reader is given just a brief overview of each approach. We hope that the clinical and empirical relevance of these models will whet the reader's appetite to delve further into learning more about them. In each chapter we identify major references for additional reading. Of course, no one can learn therapy—brief, dynamic, or otherwise—solely from books. We therefore encourage readers to also obtain clinical supervision in the particular approaches in order to practice them with sophistication and satisfaction.

■ REFERENCES

Bauer GP, Kobos JC: Brief Therapy: Short-Term Psychodynamic Intervention. Northvale, NJ, Jason Aronson, 1987

Bloom BL: Planned Short-Term Psychotherapy, 2nd Edition. Boston, MA, Allyn and Bacon, 1997

Bloom BL: Focused single-session psychotherapy: a review of the clinical and research literature. Brief Treatment and Crisis Intervention 1:75–86, 2001

Bolter K, Levenson H, Alvarez W: Differences in values between short-term and long-term therapists. Prof Psychol Res Pr 4:285–290, 1990

Budman SH, Gurman AS: Theory and Practice of Brief Psychotherapy. New York, Guilford, 1988

Burlingame GM, Fuhriman A, Paul S, et al: Implementing a time-limited therapy program: differential effects of training and experience. Psychotherapy: Theory, Research and Practice 26:303–312, 1989

Cummings NA: The dismantling of our health system: strategies for the survival of psychological practice. Am Psychol 41:426–431, 1986

Davidovitz D, Levenson H: National survey on practice and training in brief therapy: comparison of psychologists, psychiatrists and social workers. Paper presented at the annual meeting of the American Psychological Association, New York, August 1995

Gabbard GO: Psychodynamic Psychiatry in Clinical Practice, 3rd Edition. Washington, DC, American Psychiatric Press, 2000

Howard KI, Kopta SM, Krause MS, et al: The dose-effect relationship in psychotherapy. Am Psychol 41:159–164, 1986

Hoyt MF: Therapist resistances to short-term dynamic psychotherapy. J Am Acad Psychoanal 13:93–112, 1985

Koss MP, Shiang J: Research on brief psychotherapy, in Handbook of Psychotherapy and Behavior Change, 4th Edition. Edited by Bergin AE, Garfield SL. New York, Wiley, 1993, pp. 664–700

Levenson H, Burg J: Training psychologists in the era of managed care, in A Psychologist's Proactive Guide to Managed Mental Health Care. Edited by Kent AJ, Hersen M. Mahwah, NJ, Erlbaum, 2000, pp. 113–140

Levenson H, Davidovitz D: Brief therapy prevalence and training: a national survey of psychologists. Psychotherapy 37:335–340, 2000

Levenson H, Strupp HH: Recommendations for the future of training in brief dynamic psychotherapy. J Clin Psychol 55:385–391, 1999

Levenson H, Speed J, Budman SH: Therapist's experience, training, and skill in brief therapy: a bicoastal survey. Am J Psychother 49:95–117, 1995

Levenson H, Butler SF, Bein E: Brief dynamic individual psychotherapy, in The American Psychiatric Press Textbook of Psychiatry, 4th Edition. Edited by Hales RE, Yudofsky SC, Talbott JA. Washington, DC, American Psychiatric Publishing, in press

Marrow AJ: The Practical Theorist. New York, Basic Books, 1969

Martin ES, Schurtman R: Termination anxiety as it affects the therapist. Psychotherapy 22:92–96, 1985.

Messer SB, Warren S: Models of Brief Psychodynamic Therapy: A Comparative Approach. New York, Guilford, 1995

Mohl PC, Lomax J, Tasman A, et al: Psychotherapy training for the psychiatrist of the future. Am J Psychiatry 147:7–13, 1990

Olinsky DE, Howard KI: United and diversity among psychotherapies: a comparative perspective, in Comprehensive Textbook of Psychotherapy. Edited by Bongar B, Beutler LE. New York, Oxford University Press, 1995, pp 3–23

O'Malley SS, Foley SH, Watkins SD, et al: Therapist competence and patient outcome in interpersonal psychotherapy of depression. J Consult Clin Psychol 56:469–501, 1988

Peake TH, Bordin CM, Archer RP: Brief Psychotherapies: Changing Frames of Mind. Beverly Hills, CA, Sage, 1988

Pekarik G, Wierzbicki M: The relationship between clients' expected and actual treatment duration. Psychotherapy 23:532–534, 1986

Rounsaville BJ, O'Malley S, Folwy S, et al: Role of manual-guided training in the conduct and efficacy of interpersonal psychotherapy for depression. J Consult Clin Psychol 56:681–688, 1988

Siegel DJ: The Developing Mind: Toward a Neurobiology of Interpersonal Experience. New York, Guilford, 1999

Sifneos PE: Short-Term Dynamic Psychotherapy: Evaluation and Technique, 2nd Edition. New York, Plenum, 1987

Sullivan HS: The Interpersonal Theory of Psychiatry. New York, WW Norton, 1953

SUPPORTIVE THERAPY: TREATMENT FOR LOWER-FUNCTIONING PATIENTS... AND OTHERS?

From the time he developed psychoanalysis to the end of his life, Freud was preoccupied with the criticism that psychoanalysis was merely suggestion. Consequently, much of his writing reflects his insistence that true psychoanalysis was "gold," as compared with the "copper" of suggestion (Freud 1919/1955). This legacy in psychoanalysis led to an emphasis on the more expressive and technical aspects of psychoanalysis.

In traditional psychoanalysis, the patient engages in free association, saying anything and everything that comes to mind, while the quiet, listening analyst attempts to maintain a neutral stance. This neutrality was intended to prevent the analyst from revealing much about himself or herself. In the absence of information about the therapist, the patient's reactions to the therapist were expected to reflect, in a more or less pure fashion, the patient's conflicts with significant others in his or her past.

The resulting relationship was highly artificial and could be quite awkward and uncomfortable for patients. Consider, for instance, the practice of some analysts to refuse to answer questions. Were the patient to ask, "Are you married?" the analyst might answer, "Do you think I am married?" or "Does it matter if I am married?" The tension and anxiety that resulted from such stilted

---

Consider this approach for patients who:

Demonstrate some degree of ego deficit or insufficiency; that is, they

- Are unable to be introspective
- Are alexithymic—meaning that they have difficulty naming, discussing, and modulating emotions (aggression can be a particular problem in patients for whom supportive therapy is suitable)
- Are unable to tolerate painful emotions and suffering
- Have poor object relations and lack the capacity for mutuality and reciprocity
- Make prominent use of primitive defenses, such as projection, denial, and splitting
- Have difficulty trusting others
- May tend to somaticize rather than to experience problems
- Are unable to deal with, acknowledge, or productively discuss transference

---

Source. Adapted from the discussion of supportive therapy by Pinsker et al. (1991).

---

interaction supposedly brought to the fore fantasy material to be interpreted. The goal was to make the unconscious conscious and to change the patient's personality structure.

The extremely rigid and restrictive stance of tradition has given way, even in psychoanalysis, to more flexibility and naturalness (Gabbard 1990). Expressive techniques are still designed to bring into the patient's conscious awareness thoughts, feelings, and patterns of behavior of which he or she was hitherto unaware. This remains an anxiety-provoking experience and requires a patient who is very actively involved. A patient in expressive therapy must be willing and able to cooperate with the therapist in an admittedly peculiar interaction. The ability to acknowledge and discuss feelings and to invest at least some minimal level of trust in the therapist is essential for any expressive exploration. Finally, the defining technique of dynamic psychotherapy, namely, working with the patient's transference, requires the patient to be able to set aside his or her immediate feelings—for instance, of anger—and to consider how feelings toward the therapist might illuminate conflicts with others in the patient's current and past life.

Obviously, patients vary in their willingness and ability to engage in such a stylized interaction. Some patients (including therapists in therapy) can clearly engage in and benefit from anxiety-provoking techniques. Therapists have referred to these "ideal" patients as YAVIS (young, attractive, verbal, intelligent, and sophisticated). Other patients are essentially unable to participate in such a relationship. What, then, does dynamic therapy have to offer to these people?

As Luborsky (1984) has pointed out in his classic manual on supportive-expressive therapy, most psychotherapies, even the most expressive, have supportive components. Luborsky argues that patient characteristics determine the appropriate proportions of supportiveness versus expressiveness. The greater the psychiatric severity, the more supportive and less expressive the therapy may be. We tend to agree with Luborsky in this regard and believe that a predominantly supportive therapy can be a very effective and helpful treatment for many patients. In this chapter, we discuss therapy directed primarily toward the supportive end of the supportive-expressive continuum. However, given the increasing demand that therapy for all patients be extremely brief (six to eight sessions), the techniques of supportive therapy may become more in evidence, regardless of the functional status or psychotherapy potential of the patient.

Our presentation here relies greatly on the work of Pinsker et al. (1991) at the Beth Israel Psychotherapy Research Program to characterize the specific techniques of supportive psychotherapy. These authors have made a contribution by articulating components of psychotherapy that have long been ignored in the psychodynamic literature, despite the fact that supportive therapy remains the kind of treatment that is most likely to be provided to most psychiatric patients in this country.

■ DEFINITION OF SUPPORTIVE PSYCHOTHERAPY

In contrast to the overall objective of expressive psychotherapy, namely, to bring about personality change, Pinsker et al. (1991) define supportive psychotherapy in this way:

> Individual dynamic supportive psychotherapy is a dyadic treatment characterized by use of direct measures to ameliorate symptoms and to maintain, restore, or improve self-esteem, adaptive skills, and ego function. (p. 221)

Such a definition does not rule out the therapist's attention to transference issues. The therapist continues to monitor "allusions to the transference" (see Chapter 5) as a way of monitoring and managing the state of the patient-therapist relationship. Appropriate transference gratification is another hallmark of supportive therapy (Rockland 1989). Finally, in contrast to more expressive therapy, the major focus of supportive therapy is the patient's current circumstances. The focus of supportive therapy is often on the immediate problems that have brought the patient to treatment. Thus, treatment for a patient who is chronically depressed does not focus on securing changes to elements within the personality that contribute to the chronic depression, but rather on ameliorating the current deterioration in functioning and returning the patient to his or her baseline. Although this goal may appear to be modest, our experience and some empirical work (e.g., Piper et al. 1998, 1999) suggest that one should not underestimate the power of supportive interventions for patients' long-term adjustment.

■ SELECTION OF PATIENTS

Although there is little controversy regarding the use of supportive techniques with low-functioning patients, therapists have been less comfortable with the use of supportive techniques for higher-functioning patients, for whom expressive therapy has been the traditional treatment of choice (Pinsker et al. 1991). It is our opinion that the responsible therapist must take a practical stand, holding the interests of the patient as the paramount deciding factor. Rather than relying solely on patient characteristics, it is vital to take into account the resources available for the current round of therapy.

For a talented patient who is interested in personality exploration and change and who has the resources, a decidedly expressive therapy approach is warranted. Indeed, as is discussed in Chapter 5 ("Time-Limited Dynamic Psychotherapy"), much can be done with a willing patient in a relatively brief period (20–25 sessions). Some patients, however, have very limited insurance coverage, and it may be most responsible for the therapist to focus, in a supportive way, on the immediate concerns that have brought that patient to therapy, regardless of the patient's potential for therapy. This blurs further the traditional demarcation between patients who are suitable for the gold of expressive therapy and the lower-functioning, ego-deficit patients who must make do with the so-called inferior copper of supportive therapy.

■ GOALS OF TREATMENT

Setting explicit goals is of central importance for supportive therapy, as is true of all approaches to relatively brief treatment. Coming to an agreement on an agenda for treatment permits the patient to have a sense of control in the relationship and can reduce anxiety by making the therapeutic process less uncertain and less unfocused. Often the patient clearly articulates the overall goal by a statement such as "I want to stop being depressed." It is the therapist's job to formulate the dynamics of the patient's symptoms or current difficulties and to begin to make connections with issues such as self-esteem and adaptive functioning. The therapist should be able to convey the connections between the issues to be discussed and the patient's overall goals, which must be realistic. Rather than a total elimination of symptomatology in a chronically symptomatic patient, Pinsker et al. (1991) recommend goals such as the following:

- The patient should acquire the ability to understand the connection between his or her problems and poor self-esteem and/or lack of adaptive skills.
- The patient should understand how various symptoms, behaviors, or feelings are manifestations of his or her problems with self-esteem and poor adaptive skills.
- The patient should gain control of strategies for coping with his or her problems.

Change, therefore, is not the result of resolution of unconscious conflicts. Rather, change arises from learning and through identification with an "accepting, well-related therapist" (Pinsker et al. 1991, p. 226). Supportive therapy seeks to improve patients' lives by directly striving for improved self-esteem and acquisition of better adaptive skills. Poor self-esteem tends to be associated with helplessness, demoralization, and an unwillingness to try new ways of dealing with problems. In the context of a good (though uninterpreted) relationship with a therapist, the patient's self-esteem can improve, increasing openness to learning new skills. Rather than attempting to remove defenses through interpretation, supportive therapy strives to correct distorted perceptions of self and others through education. In summary, the good outcome in supportive therapy is "increased self-esteem, reduction in experienced anxiety or dysphoria, and a resultant stabilization or increase in adaptive functioning" (Pinsker et al. 1991, p. 227).

■ THE THERAPEUTIC ALLIANCE

Considerable psychotherapy research confirms the central place of the therapeutic alliance in achieving a positive outcome (Henry et al. 1994). In supportive therapy, the role of the therapeutic alliance is especially emphasized and is enhanced through the use of accurate empathic responses, validation of feeling states, a respectful and warm attitude, reassurance, and other overt and conventional efforts to establish a good relationship. Positive transference is not interpreted but is accepted as evidence that a positive alliance is developing.

Negative transference can threaten the therapeutic alliance, and the therapist must be alert to its emergence. With higher-functioning patients, detailed examination and clarification of the negative feelings and identification of their source can be constructive. This approach, however, requires that patients possess the skills to separate the negative feelings from the immediate interpersonal context and to examine those feelings. To explore and talk about strong, negative feelings with the person to whom those feelings are directed is a very high-level skill that certain patients may simply be unable to perform. With lower-functioning patients, the therapist should consider changing his or her stance, as one might when talking with someone who is becoming angry or distant in a social setting.

■ TECHNIQUES OF SUPPORTIVE THERAPY

In this section we present a list of the techniques outlined by Pinsker et al. (1991), who present these technical considerations as applicable to both lower- and higher-functioning patients. Therapy with markedly impaired patients is more likely to involve the use of direct measures to improve self-esteem and functioning. Reassurance, praise, encouragement, and direct advice are examples of such direct measures, the goal of which is to develop more adaptive coping strategies and to contain symptoms. Higher-functioning patients are more likely to spend time examining relationships, self-concept issues, and patterns of feeling and behaving.

Reducing Anxiety

The stance of the therapist is designed to reduce uncertainty and the anxiety that usually accompanies it. Patients who are beginning therapy are asked to open up in an unfamiliar and possibly threatening setting. The individual who may resist opening up to an intimate is now asked to spill all to a virtual stranger—in the stranger's office, on his or her turf. Such a patient may have thoughts such as "What could happen here? Will the therapist laugh at me or ridicule me? What if I talk about the wrong topic? What if I sound stupid?"

Such concerns are particularly likely to inhibit insecure individuals seeking therapy.

The supportive therapy approach is to adopt a conversational style of relating to patients. This does not mean that the discussion is like ordinary conversation, because the therapist never takes the floor. However, appropriate questions are generally answered, a comment might be offered just to show that the therapist is listening, and interjections and comments are made as they might be in an ordinary social conversation in which one person is intent on hearing and understanding what the other person is saying. The therapist should avoid challenging or provoking the patient and should never make pronouncements such as "You feel such and such." It is often wise to couch an observation in qualifiers that allow the patient an out. People generally respond well to an empathic, curious attitude on the part of an active listener.

Anxiety is also further reduced by increasing the patient's sense of control. One way to do this is for the therapist to explain what "we" are doing, allowing the patient to be prepared for what will happen. If the therapist is about to say something that might upset a patient, warning the patient that what is about to be said might be upsetting helps give the patient a measure of control, as does asking if the patient is willing to go on. This is analogous to informing patients of what comes next during a physical examination. The therapist should always be patient and respectful and should back off if the patient requests it or becomes upset.

Enhancing Self-Esteem

Many patients feel that they are to blame for their problems. They are sure that the world will judge them. Indeed, they typically judge themselves very harshly and readily expect others, including the therapist, to judge and reject them as well. With higher-functioning patients, it is useful to draw out such a pattern, especially in the transference, and point out, for instance, how their expectation of judgment and rejection obstructs their awareness that others do not, in fact, judge or reject them. A similar dynamic may apply to lower-functioning patients, but they may be less able to recognize their ability to change such a pattern. With these patients, it may be more productive to empathize with the difficulties they have experienced. An example might be to say, "It must have been hard feeling rejected by your father." (Some therapists—for example, Mann—use empathizing with difficulties faced by higher-functioning patients to foster nondefensive collaboration; see Chapter 3.)

It is particularly important to avoid criticism and to recognize that a patient with low self-esteem is hypersensitive to criticism. Naturally, if one feels bad about oneself, it is easy to imagine that others see oneself in the same way. The therapist should be aware, however, that this can present nearly impossible dilemmas. It is difficult to find a way to talk about improving something in someone's life without the implication that he or she has done something wrong. This quandary can be addressed directly with higher-functioning patients. With lower-functioning patients, it often best, as described above, to focus on the empathic response. Statements that most people, even the self-critical, can accept are those that merely observe their criticism of themselves, such as "You are really hard on yourself" or "It sounds like you don't often give yourself a break."

Finally, patients with low self-esteem often overemphasize their negative traits and underemphasize their positive qualities and accomplishments. Especially with lower-functioning patients, it is vital to explore their history for competencies and accomplishments. Pointing out such accomplishments and competencies must be done in a genuine way; everyone has some area of competency that can be highlighted. The importance of being genuine cannot be overstated. Expert at minimizing any accomplishment, patients with low self-esteem will be on the lookout for any insincerity.

Respecting Defenses

In supportive therapy, adaptive defenses and the patient's personal style are generally respected. Defenses such as repression, reaction formation, rationalization, and intellectualization are generally encouraged, or at least are not challenged. When adaptive, denial, too, is compatible with good emotional health. Respect for the patient's defenses means, in part, not challenging them from the outset. The patient who says, "I don't want to think about it," may be expressing how he or she adaptively deals with a particular topic. A follow-up such as "Does it work to avoid thinking about it?" gives the patient a chance to consider the effectiveness of the defense.

Supportive therapy does not encourage what are considered to be maladaptive or pathological defenses. Regression is typically not an adaptive response to life's problems. Defenses such as projection, splitting, maladaptive denial, and grossly unrealistic planning should be confronted. Some lower-functioning patients, for instance, deny that they have mental problems that require medication. One low-functioning patient decided to apply for a position as a "Bosnian mercenary." Such defenses are rarely adaptive.

The admonition to respect the patient's defenses remains, however, even with unacceptable defenses. A defense is so named because it serves some psychic purpose. Ignoring this fact will lead to therapeutic failure. The therapist should always avoid arguing with the patient. It may be useful for the therapist to tell the patient that he or she is concerned and does not understand how not taking medication will help. The exploration should always be respectful of the purpose the defense serves, even if it is not immediately apparent.

Clarification, Confrontation, and Interpretation

Clarification, confrontation, and interpretation are technical maneuvers that are also an integral part of expressive therapy. In supportive therapy, however, the purpose is not to make the unconscious conscious. Clarification is used to summarize, paraphrase, and organize the patient's statements without elaboration or inference. Clarification provides evidence that the therapist is listening and understands what the patient is communicating. It can be used to improve the patient's understanding of the situation. Confrontation brings to the patient's attention something the patient is avoiding or not attending to. In supportive therapy, this is usually conducted in a specific context, like increasing some adaptive skill. Even the most supportive therapy has the goal of increasing the patient's understanding of behavior patterns that are causing ongoing problems. Confrontation around projective blaming of others—for instance, rationalizing inactivity, denied anger, or an unrealistic sense of entitlement—might help the patient sort out cause-and-effect connections that account for some of his or her problems. In this context, interpretations generally refer to making explicit the connections elicited by clarification and confrontations.

The tone and style of such a discussion are important. In anxiety-provoking expressive therapy, a patient's chronic vagueness might be challenged. In supportive therapy, a vague patient might be urged to be more specific. As Pinsker et al. (1991) point out, the goal of supportive therapy is not to explore the motivation underlying a personality style such as vagueness, but rather to facilitate the patient's ability to communicate more effectively. Interpretations that make reference to primitive, libidinal impulses are never warranted.

Rationalization

Although rationalization is a defense, not a technique, Pinsker et al. (1991) list it as one of the tools that can be used by a supportive therapist. Rationalization is a common way in which people explain why they end up doing the things they do and not doing other things. Rationalization accounts for actions (or lack of actions) without necessarily providing an understanding of the "true" motivation that might be uncovered during formal psychoanalysis.

For example, consider the decision to go to medical school. A young man might overcome some ambivalence by rationalizing that becoming a physician is a respected and well-paid profession. In psychoanalysis, however, it could emerge that his "true" motivation is an oedipal wish to "beat" and humiliate a harsh father by attaining greater social and economic status than he did, along with the wish to gain the admiration of the mother that the father could never gain.

A historical bias has favored a psychoanalytic insistence on uncovering one's "true" motivations. As a result, therapists have been reluctant to foster rationalization or any other defense. More modern approaches recognize that some defenses can be used therapeutically. In the above example, if the young man's uncomfortable ambivalence is resolved with rationalization, perhaps this is enough understanding. As with all psychotherapeutic techniques, the use of rationalization cannot be superficial. Any rationalization that is offered must hold personal meaning for the particular patient in order to be effective.

Reframing

Pinsker et al. (1991) list reframing as a useful technique to help patients improve their self-esteem and adapt more effectively. Reframing can allow the patient to see an issue from a different perspective that, in turn, permits new and different actions and ways of looking at the issue.

Consider, for instance, the case of a young man referred to treatment for violating his wife's restraining order. Exploration reveals that his increasing frustration is an extension of the control he desired to have in the relationship. Although he is unable to directly acknowledge and work with his pathological need to control others, he is responsive to a reframing of his need to regain control by staying away from his wife. He is thus able to see that violating the restraining order is not increasing his control of the situation. Instead, as the police and courts increasingly take her side, he is steadily losing more and more control of the situation. Reframing his adherence to the restraining order as a method of gaining control permits the therapist to help this patient adopt a more adaptive coping strategy. Thus, although the personality pathology is not directly addressed, the patient is able to obey the restraining order and stay away from his wife.

Encouragement

Encouragement, reassurance, and praise are ways in which people support each other. Stereotypic views of dynamic therapy have resulted in many therapists being reluctant to "flatter the patient" or to "feed the narcissism" (Viederman 1989, p. 151). Supporting self-esteem and adaptive coping, however, is an integral part of support-ive therapy.

Although praise may reinforce certain behaviors, such encour-agement or praise should not be confused with the operant behav-iorist's use of praise as a reinforcer. In dynamically oriented supportive therapy, praise and encouragement are not used to reinforce certain behaviors. Rather, praise and encouragement should be genuine ex-pressions from the therapist that will communicate goodwill to the patient and facilitate the therapeutic alliance. As this implies, praise must be based on facts and directed toward something the patient considers meaningful. Insincere or manipulative praise will be de-tected by the patient and may foster suspicion that the therapist is presenting a false front. Such a perception runs the risk of damaging rather than strengthening the alliance.

Reassurance also has the direct effect of reducing anxiety. However, this, too, must be expressed in terms that are meaningful to the patient and should always be based on fact. Reassurance should not unrealistically promise that things will get better, and the therapist should stick to areas of expertise or knowledge. Reassur-ance on some situation for which the therapist has no real insight (e.g., legal concerns) is unlikely to be reassuring.

In general, the use of overt encouragement, praise, and reas-surance should probably be used sparingly. Such direct positive statements can be very effective coming from a therapist or other authority figure, such as a physician. This impact stems in part from the fact that such statements are unexpected. Overuse of such state-ments will dilute the impact and, at worst, may create concerns in the patient's mind about the therapist's sincerity. A therapist whose credibility is lost will be ineffective.

Advising

Giving advice is something that many therapists learn explicitly not to do. Indeed, there are good reasons to avoid giving advice, the most important of which is that most people with problems typi-cally receive all kinds of advice from family and friends. In most cases, the primary service that a therapist has to offer is to listen and reflect; that is, the therapist should do what other people do not do.

The prohibition against offering advice can be modified for lower-functioning patients. Certain patients have trouble with virtually every aspect of daily life, and some of these areas may fall within the scope of therapy. Pinsker et al. (1991) suggest that advice is relevant if it is designed to help the patient act in ways that will enhance self-esteem, improve adaptive skills, or improve ego functioning. They recommend that the basis and rationale for any advice should be stated. Thus, a statement such as "You should work" should be avoided in favor of something like "Most people who stop working don't feel better—not working protects you from some stress, but it's usually bad for self-esteem." As with encouragement, praise, and reassurance, the therapist should be speaking as an expert, not as an authority.

Rehearsal or Anticipation

A technique that can help patients deal effectively with new and stressful situations is to anticipate and rehearse such situations. In the safety of the therapist's office, patients can rehearse what they want to say to, for example, a boss about some reprimand or during a necessary meeting with an abusive ex-spouse. Patients can run through some future event and thereby reduce the anticipatory anxiety associated with such events. Rehearsal further allows patients to directly adopt and practice new and unfamiliar coping strategies. It also can provide a forum for discussing their anticipated reactions or various approaches they might take. For instance, rehearsing a job interview with a very shy patient can reveal to both the patient and the therapist the patient's expectation of failure and the influence of this on how he or she comes across in the interview situation.

Responding to Ventilation

In a sense, one of the most valuable services that verbal therapies offer is the opportunity for an individual to ventilate. Reflection will confirm that there are really very few times in ordinary social intercourse when one can sit with another person and get it all off one's chest. Many times, patients bring to therapy a sad or traumatic story that they have never been able to really tell anyone. By actively listening, the therapist can deepen the experience of ventilation. Such active responses include tracking (making comments or asking questions that show the therapist is following the patient's story), universalizing (making it clear that many people have similar feelings, wishes, or problems), and decatastrophizing (identifying where a patient may have exaggerated problems or issues and offer a more proportioned interpretation).

Attention to, Not Interpretation of, Transference

Transference holds a central position in the theory and practice of dynamic psychotherapy. What distinguishes dynamic supportive therapy from any other version of supportive therapy is the recognition that transference affects the patient's communications. This is as true for lower-functioning patients as it is for higher-functioning patients. Toward the expressive end of the continuum, allusions to the transference lead to exploration and possibly interpretation. Toward the supportive end, such allusions from lower-functioning patients inform the therapist about what is on the patient's mind but is difficult for him or her to articulate. These insights can help the therapist guide the discussion, but these allusions generally should not be explored as they would be in expressive therapy. In the following case example, the therapist detects a rather extreme allusion to the transference from a young schizophrenic man.

Case Example

A therapist has been working with a schizophrenic man for about 2 years, on both an inpatient and an outpatient basis. The therapist is now moving to another part of the country. During their last session, the schizophrenic man begins the session by saying:

Patient: I'm a banana.
Therapist: Tell me about bananas.

Patient: They hang around all day and don't do anything all day long.

Therapist: Anything else?

Patient: You take off their skin and eat what's inside. When you're done with them, you throw them away.

Therapist: It's hard that I'm leaving, isn't it?

Patient: Yeah, that's it. I don't know who I'll have to talk to.

This low-functioning patient, who was not actively psychotic at the moment, was having feelings that he could not express. His "banana" comment is at first indecipherable but with some questioning emerges clearly as an allusion to thoughts and feelings about the therapist that he had difficulty expressing. The therapist used the insight gained from the realization that the comment referred to what was happening in the here and now and was able to move the conversation quickly in a more overt and productive direction.

Conclusion

The supportive techniques outlined here and listed in Table 2–1 are presented for use largely with lower-functioning patients. However, these techniques are equally suitable for higher-functioning patients, especially in a very brief therapy format. Such techniques are good adjuncts to any therapeutic stance or approach.

The experienced therapist knows, however, that techniques, in and of themselves, are not supportive or even effective. The effect of any particular technical maneuver is a direct result of the meaning that technique has for the individual patient (Butler and Strupp 1986). What one patient experiences as supportive another might see as condescending, manipulative, or negative in some other way.

For example, two patients might successfully complete some task like registering for a class. One might easily accept praise for this from the therapist, whereas the other reacts with shame, saying in essence, "Anyone should be able to register for a class." The therapist who assumes that praise, or any particular technique, is universally supportive will miss important information. Tracking such reactions to what the therapist does is a vital skill for any therapist.

TABLE 2–1.   **Techniques of supportive dynamic psychotherapy**

Reducing anxiety

Enhancing self-esteem

Respecting defenses

Clarification, confrontation, and interpretation

Rationalization

Reframing

Encouragement

Advising

Rehearsal or anticipation

Responding to ventilation

Attention to, not interpretation of, transference

Source.   Adapted from Pinsker et al. 1991.

The following vignette is excerpted from the work of Pinsker et al. (1991) and illustrates some supportive techniques.

■ CLINICAL ILLUSTRATION

The patient is a young woman who began treatment because she was depressed and felt dissatisfied with her life. As therapy has progressed, it has become clear that she judges herself as indecisive and uncertain about everything. In this session, the patient discussed having taken a second job, a night job at a bar, which she quit after a few days.

> Patient: At first I felt bad to start and quit. It wasn't as good as I thought it was going to be, and I was very tired the next day. It's more important I do well at my regular job.
>
> Therapist [*clarifies*]: You felt bad about quitting, but only a little bad.
>
> Patient: Yeah. I felt a little bad because I could make money if I stuck it out, but I realized it was going to be hard. If people stayed late, I'd have to stay, too. And they wanted me to work on nights when I had school.
>
> Therapist [*asks for confirmation of his understanding of the patient's statements*]: Well, would I be correct if I said that

you still think an extra job to make some money is a good idea, but that this is not the way to do it?

Patient: I just realized I didn't have time for school. The best thing about it is that now I value my time more. After that, now my schedule seems great.

Therapist [*fact-based praise*]: Well, you made this decision without a lot of uncertainty.

Patient: No, I was pretty sure.

Therapist [*asks for feedback about accuracy of praise*]: It sounds to me like taking the job was a reasonable thing to do, and getting out as soon as you saw that it wasn't good was also a reasonable thing to do. Would you agree?

Patient: Yeah.

Therapist [*reminds patient of their agenda and attempts to enhance self-esteem by reinforcing patient's awareness of good adaptive function*]: Since I'm always coming back to the issue of self-confidence—what did it do for your self-confidence that you made a decision to do it and then you made a decision to stop doing it?

Patient: Yeah, it was OK. At first I thought I was copping out because I didn't think I'd be able to handle it, but by the third night, I was catching on...so last week was a tough week.

Therapist [*makes empathic conversational response*]: It sure sounds like it!

This short vignette illustrates the use of some of the techniques described in this chapter. Note the cautious way in which the therapist phrases his questions, which reflects his attempt to not take anything for granted. The goal is to gain an understanding of what the patient is saying that is as complete as possible. The therapist also demonstrates how to check in with the patient after using a technique such as praise to ensure that he and the patient agree on the meaning of what has just transpired.

■ EMPIRICAL FINDINGS

Until recently, supportive therapy was not considered a separate kind of therapy. As discussed earlier, most of the focus in dynamic therapy is on expressive therapy, making the assumption that supportive therapy could certainly be done by an accomplished expressive therapist. In general, psychotherapy research shows that the quality of the therapeutic alliance tends to be associated with outcome (Winston et al. 1986). Supportive techniques have been shown to be at least as helpful as drugs or other therapies, such as cognitive, behavioral, or insight-oriented therapies, in patients with coronary artery disease (Razin 1982), opiate addiction (Woody et al. 1983), phobia (Klein et al. 1983), and "anxious depression" (Schwab 1984). The value of supportive therapy has been supported in a study of treatment for chronic schizophrenia (Carpenter 1984) and a study of severely disturbed, nonpsychotic patients conducted over 40 years at the Menninger Clinic (Wallerstein 1989). In both studies, contrary to expectations, supportive therapy was found to be at least as effective as expressive methods, and in some cases was more so. Pinsker and colleagues (Rosenthal et al. 1999) found that supportive therapy improved patients' interpersonal functioning. It should be noted, however, that many of these latter studies of supportive therapy did not involve brief therapies, at least by today's standards. The study by Rosenthal et al. (1999) was relatively brief but was about 40 sessions long.

Piper and colleagues (W. E. Piper, H. F. A. Azim, A. S. Joyce, and M. McCallum, "Manual for Time-Limited, Short-Term Individual Therapies: Interpretive and Supported Forms," unpublished data, June 1993) produced a manual outlining both interpretative and supportive therapy techniques and studied therapies that were about 20 sessions long (a typical length for a brief, dynamic therapeutic approach). The supportive approach is similar to the one outlined in this chapter; that is, the primary objective is to improve patients' immediate adaptation to their life situation. Anxiety and regression in the session are minimized, and the therapist provides praise and immediate gratification. The therapist's stance is active, noninterpretive, and focused on patients' current external relationships (Piper et al 1998).

In clinical trials comparing interpretive and supportive therapies (Piper et al. 1998, 1999), supportive therapy produced significant improvements in patient outcomes and outcomes that were comparable to those obtained by the interpretative therapies. Indeed, supportive therapy produced significantly fewer dropouts (6.3%) than did interpretive therapy (23.4%). Not surprisingly, patients who did best in interpretive therapy had a higher quality of object relations, meaning they had a history of satisfactory give-and-take relationships that may have made them more able to tolerate the demands of interpretive therapy. Supportive therapy, on the other hand, was much less sensitive to this patient characteristic, so that patients with both higher and lower levels of object relational quality did well in this 20-session therapy.

These data suggest that, although perhaps very talented patients with extensive resources may benefit from longer-term expressive or interpretative therapies, supportive therapy may be highly suitable for most patients in a brief format. Furthermore, the research generally confirms the position expressed in this chapter that severely disturbed patients are more likely to respond to supportive rather than expressive techniques.

■ RELEVANCE FOR MANAGED CARE

A time frame for brief, supportive therapy has been set at about 40 sessions by the Beth Israel Psychotherapy Research Program. Today, a time frame of 40 sessions may not be possible because many managed care organizations often limit outpatient sessions to 20 or fewer. Research by Piper and colleagues (1998, 1999) clearly demonstrates that supportive therapy can be quite effective for patients in a 20-session format. Our impression is that many of the techniques of supportive therapy outlined in this chapter can be extraordinarily useful within any number of sessions. Even in the context of a single session, techniques to reduce anxiety, enhance self-esteem, and provide clarification can be beneficial to patients in distress. The hallmark of a supportive therapist is to be flexible with what the patient offers. This stance applies not only to the patient's characteristics but also to his or her mental health coverage.

In addition to use with such lower-functioning patients, however, there is reason to believe that the techniques of supportive therapy may also be suitable for a wide range of patients in an era of very brief, highly managed care

■ REFERENCES

Butler SF, Strupp HH: "Specific" and "nonspecific" factors in psychotherapy: a problematic paradigm for psychotherapy research. Psychotherapy 23:30–40, 1986

Carpenter WT: A perspective on the psychotherapy of schizophrenia project. Schizophr Bull 10:599–603, 1984

Freud S: Line of advance in psychoanalytic therapy (1919), in The Standard Edition of the Complete Psychological Works of Sigmund Freud, Vol 17. Translated and edited by Strachey J. London, Hogarth Press, 1955, pp 157–168

Gabbard GO: Psychodynamic Psychiatry in Clinical Practice. Washington, DC, American Psychiatric Press, 1990

Henry WP, Strupp HH, Schacht TE, et al: Psychodynamic approaches, in Handbook of Psychotherapy and Behavior Change, 4th Edition. Edited by Bergin AE, Garfield SL. New York, Wiley, 1994, pp 467–508

Klein DF, Zitrin CM, Woerner MG, et al: Treatment of phobias: behavior therapy and supportive psychotherapy: are there any specific ingredients? Arch Gen Psychiatry 40:139–145, 1983

Luborsky L: Principles of Psychoanalytic Psychotherapy: A Manual for Supportive-Expressive Treatment. New York, Basic Books, 1984

Pinsker H, Rosenthal R, McCullough L: Dynamic supportive therapy, in Handbook of Short-Term Dynamic Psychotherapy. Edited by Crits-Christoph P, Barber JP. New York, Basic Books, 1991, pp 220–247

Piper WE, Joyce AS, McCallum M, et al: Interpretative and supportive forms of psychotherapy and patient personality variables. J Consult Clin Psychol 66:558–567, 1998

Piper WE, McCallum M, Joyce AS, et al: Follow-up findings for interpretative and supportive forms of psychotherapy and patient personality variables. J Consult Clin Psychol 67:267–273, 1999

Razin AM: Psychosocial intervention in coronary artery disease: a review. Psychosom Med 44:363–387, 1982

Rockland LH: Supportive Therapy: A Psychodynamic Approach. New York, Basic Books, 1989

Rosenthal RN, Muran JC, Pinsker H, et al: Interpersonal change in brief supportive psychotherapy. J Psychother Pract Res 8:55–63, 1999

Schwab JJ: Anxiety and depression. Clin Ther 6:536–545, 1984

Viederman M: The active dynamic interview and the supportive relationship. Compr Psychiatry 25:147–157, 1989

Wallerstein RS: The psychotherapy research project of the Menninger Foundation: an overview. J Consult Clin Psychol 57:195–205, 1989

Winston A, Pinsker H, McCullough L: A review of supportive psychotherapy. Hosp Community Psychiatry 37:1105–1114, 1986

Woody GE, Luborsky L, McLellan AT, et al: Psychotherapy for opiate addicts. Natl Inst Drug Abuse Res Monogr Ser 43:59–70, 1983

3

TIME-LIMITED THERAPY

■ BASIC FRAMEWORK

Birth ——————————— **Death**

Focus on the line above from birth to death. Place an × where you think you are at the present time.

Now you are in the perfect frame of mind to comprehend Mann's model of time-limited psychotherapy (TLP) (Mann 1973; Mann and Goldman 1991). Whereas other theorists have developed brief models out of economic necessity or clinical need in an era of managed care, tightening budgets, and waiting lists, TLP is based on using the structure of finite and limited time to help the patient confront difficulties in mastering separation anxiety.

In an almost poetic opening to his book *Time-Limited Psychotherapy*, Mann (1973) describes how folklore conveys limitless time and immortality in the figure of an abundant woman, whereas time as a limited commodity is represented by Father Time, with a beard and a scythe. He further states how a sense of timelessness is a part of a person's unconscious. He contrasts child time (subjective, eternal, endless) with adult time (objective, real, clock).

The reader can readily appreciate the difference between clock time (sundial to digital) and perceived time. With the latter, there are times when we are so bored or distressed that, as the song goes, "the moments seem like hours, the hours go so slowly." At other times, usually in pleasurable situations, even days can seem to rush by in a blur.

> **Consider this approach for patients who:**
>
> - Have individuation-separation issues
> - Are young adults entering the developmental stage of identity versus role diffusion
> - Are going through a complicated bereavement
> - Have dependent-passive personality styles
> - Have an adjustment disorder due to separation or loss (e.g., of status, ability, money, power)
> - Have existential issues about the meaning of their lives

TLP is psychodynamic in its basic philosophy and technique (e.g., use of conflict, resistance, transference, and interpretation), but it has a strong existential overlay:

> Although there is no effective means for struggling against time, we do try….If one can eliminate time sense, one can also avoid the ultimate separation that time brings—death. (Mann 1973, p. 6)

Mann sees that there is one basic human dilemma revolving around conflicts with separation—individuation. On the one hand, the person desires to be in a pleasurable state of timelessness where all needs are taken care of; on the other hand, one is painfully aware that time does pass and that one needs to make his or her own way. Dysfunction occurs when people cannot master or even tolerate the sense of separateness and autonomy and continue to act as if someday they will be rescued from their present state and no longer have to confront those issues.

■ THEORY AND TECHNIQUE

TLP is built around the aphorism "process follows structure." Mann (1973) designed a time-limited structure for the therapy that ideally would activate the patient's anxiety regarding separation and loss and thus permit an examination and more successful resolution of his or her conflicts.

Any psychotherapy that is limited in time brings fresh flame to the enduring presence in all persons of the conflict between time-lessness, infinite time, immortality, and the omnipotent fantasies of childhood, on the one hand, and time, finite time, reality, and death, on the other hand. The wishes of the unconscious are timeless and promptly run counter to an offer of help in which time is limited. Thus, any time-limited psychotherapy addresses itself to both child time and adult time (Mann 1973, pp. 10–11).

Mann's model of TLP is built on a tight structure of 12 sessions. Although Mann says that the 12 sessions can be distributed on the basis of the patient's needs (e.g., a less well-functioning patient may be seen in weekly half-hour visits spread out over 24 weeks), most patients who are accepted for TLP are seen for the traditional 50-minute weekly session. (Mann admonishes practitioners not to call the 50-minute session an "hour": "This may appear to be an obsessional adherence to literalness. However, when the meaning of time is to be the lever that motivates and moves the patient, there is a sufficient mix of fantasy and reality without making for an unnecessary additional complication by calling a less than 60-minute meeting an hour" [Mann 1973, p. 16].)

To the often-asked question, "Why 12 sessions?" Mann simply states that the number 12 is somewhat arbitrary, but that "experience has demonstrated that twelve treatment sessions is probably the minimal time required for a series of dynamic events to develop, flourish, and be available for discussion, examination, and resolution" (Mann 1973, p. 15). In other words, it might take patients at least that amount of time to engage in the therapeutic relationship, experience the relationship, and then detach. Because the therapy is designed to heighten the conflicts between realistic individuation and wishful merger, it is critical for the patient to have a sense of the passage of time in which there is a beginning, a middle, and an end. Mann and Goldman (1991) point out that

...in all varieties of psychotherapy, the patient knows when therapy has begun, but he is seldom fully aware of the middle of treatment and usually does not recognize the end of treatment until the subject is explicitly discussed. In time-limited psychotherapy, the beginning, middle, and end are known from the start. (p. 10)

■ PHASES OF TREATMENT

Intake/Selection

Initially, an intake is performed, during which time historical data are obtained, the patient's psychological state is assessed, and a tentative diagnosis is given. One or two such evaluation meetings usually take place before TLP begins.

Table 3–1 lists the selection criteria for TLP. During the process of the initial interviews, the therapist ascertains a central issue or complaint. If the patient is so diffuse that such a central issue cannot be discerned, the therapist should consider the possibility of some psychotic thought process or a low motivation for change, either of which would signal that TLP is not appropriate for the patient.

Mann (1973) reasons that young men and women who developmentally are facing the pressures of adulthood are particularly well suited to the focus and process of TLP. The most critical selection criterion, however, pertains to an individual's ability to rapidly attach and detach emotionally (i.e., tolerate loss) without decompensating (e.g., returning to a less mature defense and increasing symptoms). The areas that are important to know about to ascertain a patient's suitability for TLP include how he or she has handled previous losses, the occurrence of early deprivations, the ability to relate to the interviewer, and the capacity for affective expression. Despite these specifics,

...each patient, regardless of his presenting complaint and early history, must be evaluated on his own terms without any preconceived prejudice or bias....[C]areful assessment of the patient's life history in terms of his relative success in work and in relationships with others becomes an effective means for determining suitability for time-limited psychotherapy. (Mann and Goldman 1991, pp. 61–62)

TABLE 3–1. **Selection criteria for patients receiving time-limited psychotherapy**

Inclusion criteria
    Capacity for rapid affective involvement and toleration of loss without serious disruption in functioning
    Adjustment disorders
    Neurotic character structure

Questionable status
    Obsessional characters (especially those with major defenses of isolation and intellectualization)
    Borderline patients
    Narcissistic disorders
    Psychosomatic disorders

Exclusion criteria
    Schizophrenia
    Bipolar affective disorders
    Schizoid disorders

Honeymoon Phase

The 3-month course of therapy can be conceptually divided into three phases, each approximately 1 month long. The first phase is aptly called the honeymoon. After being accepted for TLP, the patient is told that his or her therapy will last 12 sessions, spread over 3 months. Mann gives the exact date of the last meeting to the patient and even takes out his calendar to dramatically underscore the significance and definiteness of the specific date. Theoretically, the adult part of the patient understands all of these strictures and realizes that 12 sessions is not a long time. The child portion of the patient, however, has the feeling that 3 months is very far in the future. It is not unusual for patients to "forget" how many sessions they have left and even to deny that they were told that therapy was to be time limited. Sometimes, however, the patient does ask whether 12 sessions will be enough. Mann sees such a question as stemming from a combination of the wish for endless time, the realistic awareness of calendar time, and the understanding of the time-limited nature of the therapy. He advises that if TLP is appropriate for the patient, the answer to the patient's question is a simple and "genuinely confident 'yes'" (Mann 1973, p. 21).

In the honeymoon phase, the therapist is seen as the good and providing parent who will meet all needs and remedy past injustices; the therapeutic alliance is strong, positive, and unambivalent. During this phase, patients report a lessening of symptoms and an increase in hope in the process and faith in the therapist.

As early as possible, the therapist learns and then clarifies for the patient his or her central issue or major problem. Although patients usually come to therapy wanting treatment for specific symptoms (such as depression or anxiety), the TLP therapist seeks to discover the unconscious conflict that has resulted in these symptoms. To do so, the therapist must extract from the patient his or her life story, which will reveal data about the patient's past and present situation, the occurrence of difficult or traumatic events, and the ways the patient learned to respond to these painful events. The therapist is looking for repetitive events and responses that reveal the patient's typical way of handling conflict.

The therapist's statement of the patient's central issue is most helpful to the patient (i.e., can be heard more openly and less defensively) if it emphasizes how the patient has attempted to cope with the unfairness and injustices of his or her life by developing certain ways of acting and reacting. Therapists should express the patient's lifelong difficulties empathically, in terms of a "present and chronically endured pain" (i.e., recognizing that he or she has been victimized in some manner). In this way, the patient will feel supremely understood and nurtured by the therapist (further strengthening the already positive working alliance). According to TLP, this emphatic connection with the patient's pain should facilitate the patient's recognizing and processing unconscious conflicts. Table 3–2 outlines some of the ways in which the therapist can begin to ascertain the patient's central issue.

Negative Transference Phase

The second phase of treatment is the negative transference phase, which occupies the middle month of treatment. In this phase, the

---

TABLE 3–2.   **How to choose a central issue**

---

1. Listen for themes in the patient's story that are evident in the past and continue into the present.
2. Look for actions by which the patient has mastered or adapted to difficult life circumstances (usually at great personal cost).
3. Examine how the patient keeps childhood struggles and attendant adult pain out of his or her awareness.
4. Note the patient's self-image.
5. Delineate issues clustering around one of four themes:
    a. Independence versus dependence
    b. Activity versus passivity
    c. Adequate versus diminished self-esteem
    d. Unresolved or delayed grief

TLP therapist is more directive and interpretative, linking repetitive patterns with underlying conflicts. With the passage of sessions, the patient realizes that miraculous changes in his or her life situations have not occurred; he or she has not been cured. As if that weren't bad enough, the therapist is reminding the patient that the therapy is half over. Understandably, the patient reacts negatively over.

It is important during this phase for the therapist not to personalize the patient's negative reactions or to think that the therapy is going badly. In fact, it is critical from a TLP viewpoint that patients have a safe enough place to express these powerfully negative feelings that hearken back to disappointed feelings experienced (but often not expressed) with earlier (usually parental) figures in life. The therapist should invite an exploration of the patient's frustrated, ambivalent feelings, which might be overtly demonstrated through lateness, reemergence of symptoms, and outright complaints.

Termination Phase

The last, or termination, phase is critical in that it affords the patient the opportunity to separate in a less ambivalent, more mature, and more confident manner than has previously been the case. Patients will attempt to deal with the impending ending of the therapy and loss of the therapeutic relationship in their own characteristic manner, one that is typical of how they dealt with previous separations. If the therapist can deal directly and explicitly with the patient's pain and fears about ending, the patient will have a greater chance of internalizing the understanding and accepting the therapist as a replacement for earlier, disappointing parental figures:

> This time the internalization will be more positive (never totally so), less anger-laden, and less guilt-laden, thereby making separation a genuine maturational event. (Mann 1973, p. 36)

Throughout all phases of TLP, it is crucial for the therapist to stay focused on exploring the patient's central issue. In the first phase, keeping such a tight focus not only will permit a deeper understanding of those issues but also will prevent regression by restricting the scope of the work. In the middle phase, attending to the central issue keeps the patient focused despite his or her impatience—after all, from the patient's perspective, there are many important areas to discuss. This raises the patient's awareness of the conflicts embedded in the central issue—namely, that he or she, in characteristic fashion, is headed for yet another difficult separation without feeling whole. Similarly, in the last phase, the therapist discusses termination through the lens of the patient's central issue.

■ REVERBERATIONS FOR THE THERAPIST

Perhaps more than any other model of brief therapy, Mann's TLP is the most affect-laden for the therapist. Like their patients, therapists must confront their own conflicts regarding loss. In teaching this model, we have found that therapists who are inexperienced in providing brief therapy often find "very good reasons" for continuing the therapy and avoiding termination. Mann believes that it is these resistances to dealing with the separation that make for either extended, open-ended therapies or botched endings. Therapists who attempt TLP should be particularly attentive to clearly communicating the termination date to patients, avoiding ambivalent communications regarding the request for more sessions (e.g., "We'll see"), and reminding patients of the decreasing number of sessions.

■ CLINICAL ILLUSTRATION

The illustrative case example presented here (Mann and Goldman 1991) is that of Ms. A, a 40-year-old married woman with four school-age children who came for outpatient therapy because she feared she had cancer and did not have long to live. Ms. A had recently had a biopsy of a facial lesion. Although the most likely diagnosis was easily treated skin cancer, Ms. A felt that it was a surface indication of something fatal. Her history revealed multiple visits to physicians for a myriad of physical symptoms (e.g., headaches, stomach pains, burning sensations in arms and legs) for at least a decade.

In the intake interview, Ms. A indicated that she had been trained as a medical technician and was presently working in the same medical center where her father had died of a myocardial infarction at age 48. As a child, she had been concerned about his hypertension, and she talked about how she would listen for his snoring at night as a sign that he was still alive. Ms. A felt that she was a caregiver to her mother, although she acknowledged that her mother was rather independent. She was aware that she had a propensity to take care of others, which she then experienced as burdensome. Her husband seemed to be a good provider who was generally supportive of his wife of 13 years. Her earliest memory (about which she was unsure had really happened) was of being in a store with her parents at age 5 and becoming panicky when she found herself alone—abandoned.

As Ms. A continued to describe her present and past feelings and interactions with various family members, a theme emerged that she had an overpowering need to do for others while feeling unworthy herself. At the end of the first evaluation interview, Ms. A asked, "Do you think I can be helped?" to which the therapist replied, "Yes, but there is further information that I would like to have, and then I will suggest what we might do."

In the second evaluation interview, more historical information supported the therapist's hypothesis that Ms. A felt unworthy and had a compulsive need to do good for others. She would become furious with this need to constantly give with little recognition, which would in turn make her feel more guilty and undeserving. Her anger must be tied, the therapist felt, to sadistic, guilt-provoking fantasies that increased her sense of unworthiness, which in turn increased her need to be good and to do for others. In addition, she feared that if she were not good, she would be abandoned and unloved. This fear engendered anger, which mobilized guilt, which in turn was mastered by further doing good. Thus, she was trapped in this sequence of affects (Mann and Goldman 1991).

The following dialogue illustrates how the therapist empathically presented the central issue to the patient in terms of her chronically endured pain in their second meeting.[1]

> Therapist: You have always given of yourself to so many others, and yet you feel, and always have felt, both undeserving and unrewarded.
> Patient: You mean by my husband?
> Therapist: You feel unloved by him and all the others.
> Patient: I often feel that I have no friends at all.

A treatment plan of 12 sessions, with a specific ending date, focusing on the central issue was agreed to by Ms. A. Before the hour ended, she spoke about how she had no self-confidence and relayed how she was beaten with a strap by her mother.

Later in this same session, the therapist reiterated the central issue to Ms. A:

> Patient: You know, I just remember again that memory or dream, whatever it is, about my parents abandoning me in the store.

---

[1]Transcribed material is reprinted from Mann and Goldman 1991, pp. 81–98. Used with permission.

Therapist: You did to your little daughter what was done to you; you felt that you had abandoned her and you became sick.

Patient: I never thought of that.

Therapist: You have the need to be good out of fear that you will be left, unloved and uncared for.

Patient: I don't want to go on with these thoughts about myself. I feel a churning inside; my arms and face feel like they are burning.

Therapist: You are always ready to feel guilty.

The above vignette shows how the TLP therapist highlighted associative data from the patient's previous remarks to encourage her to make "intimate connections."

In the third session, the patient complained of a variety of symptoms and expressed renewed fears that she might have cancer. Her therapist reminded her of the past session, in which she did not want to talk about her fear of being abandoned.

Patient: There are times when I am afraid that my husband will leave me. I went to a meeting in which a lot of men were involved, superfluous, and depressed. I told my husband about it and I cried. He said I was making too much of it.

Therapist: You were hurt by the men and then you became angry.

Patient: Now that you mention it, I was angry with those men even before the meeting. I knew how they would act with me.

Therapist: How must a woman feel who always has to please everyone of significance to her?

Patient: Frustration.

Therapist: Anger.

Patient: I suppose I give myself very little credit for anything.

Therapist: You are very hard on yourself. For example, you must feel apprehensive and tense here because of what you must feel are my expectations of you with so little time available.

Patient: I see that and I know that I am here to do something for myself and not for you...but what has all this to do with my symptoms?

Therapist: Your symptoms serve to avoid—to keep away from your awareness—your feelings, especially angry feelings.

Patient: Why?

Therapist: Let's ignore the "why" of it at this point and instead see how you have come to an automatic way of relating— to give and give in the hope of acceptance, and inevitably you come to suffer frustration and anger—that is what we should look at further.

Patient: What about my fear that I haven't long to live?

Therapist: We will have to wait on that. I know that this is all very difficult and painful for you.

Patient: Do you still think I can be helped?

Therapist: Yes.

In this third session, the therapist again helped the patient to become aware of her feelings of anger in addition to those of hurt and frustration. The aspect of limited time was introduced. By the fourth session, the patient was feeling better—taking some risks with regard to her anger, independence, and anxiety. According to TLP, it is typical for patients to experience a decrease in symptoms during this honeymoon phase, but for this patient, a lessening of complaints may also be a manifestation of her need to please.

The week before the fifth session was "awful"; the patient had felt angry with her husband. In the session, the therapist attempted to draw out the patient's transference feelings by suggesting that perhaps Ms. A was angry with the therapist for not giving her much time. The patient told him that she would be on vacation the next week. With such planned cancellations, the therapist can simply extend the termination date by another week. If cancellations become frequent, however, the therapist should explore the patient's conflicts about ending. If the patient simply did not show up for a session, the time would not be made up.

In the sixth session, Ms. A indicated that during her vacation she had felt irritable.

Therapist: You're experiencing a good deal of anger, and it must be something that you feel toward me.

Patient: I don't see why…

Therapist: Well, you're feeling a good deal of pressure from me—so little time…

Patient: What will happen to me if I feel no better at the end and you send me on?

Therapist: How much time do we have—how many sessions left?

Patient: I don't know.

Therapist: Guess.

Patient: Five.

Therapist: No, we still have six.

Patient: The pressure of time is always there.

Therapist: The pressure of time is really the pressure that you feel from people—from me—the pressure as to whether you can do it here.

Patient: It makes me angry. I am so much more aware of being angry….

In the seventh session, the patient again underestimated the number of sessions left. Her therapist considered that this distortion was the product of her feeling that she was giving so much in the therapy and reaping so little benefit. Even if she had accurately remembered the number of sessions left, it is assumed that patients will find a way to express frustration and hopelessness midway in the therapy.

In the eighth session, the therapist reviewed with the patient how events in her life had resulted in her thinking that she was undeserving. In the ninth meeting, he interpreted to the patient that she did not want to leave him or for him to let her go. The patient agreed. In the tenth session, Ms. A talked about how she came to marry her husband.

Patient: Did I marry B out of the feeling that I had to have someone who would put me down?

Therapist: In view of your relationship with the man who preceded your husband [a man who felt superior to her], and in the light of all that we have learned, it is likely that you could not have chosen someone who would have placed you on a pedestal.

Patient: You mean this thing about being undeserving?

Therapist: Yes.
Patient: Then my relationship with my husband can change only
    by changes that I make myself?
Therapist: Yes.

As the patient continued to talk about some symptoms she had experienced during the preceding week, her therapist connected her symptoms to her feelings about her father, his illness, and her guilt about his illness. The session concluded with Ms. A asking for an evaluation of her progress to this point. The therapist thought that the patient probably wanted him to tell her that he liked her and found her worthwhile.

In the eleventh session, the therapist brought up termination, to which the patient replied that she had just come to accept the time limit and was not aware of any particular feelings toward him. She maintained this attitude until the topic of her deserving to live was raised.

Patient: I have always felt that my time is limited—that I would
    die young—and I still feel that way…(she begins to
    cry)…I'm afraid that it will all return after I'm through.
    What will I do?
Therapist: You mean then that I should not let you go.
Patient: At least if I knew I could come back to see you.
Therapist: We will talk some more about that next week.

In the last session, Ms. A, who had been relatively symptom free for 2 weeks, realized that the burning sensations in her skin happened when she was angry.

Therapist: You want me to tell you to stay?
Patient: No—I only want to know whether I can return if things
    go wrong.
Therapist: You are the kind of person who likes schedules and as-
    surances. There are no guarantees in the task of living, and
    you will have to take your chances like the rest of us. Give
    yourself some time. I think that you will do all right, and if
    you come to feel that you need help, you'll know what to do.

The therapist then recapitulated what had been learned in the therapy about Ms. A's central issue and in the last minutes reminded her to maintain her self-esteem by being vigilant about her inferiority feelings and remembering her accomplishments.

In his earlier writings, Mann (1973) indicated that it is important to have a real ending with the patient, to reinforce the idea that time is finite and that losses occur. Therefore, at the conclusion of the 12 sessions, the therapist was not supposed to see the patient again. (If the patient were not doing well at the end of the TLP, the therapist could take whatever steps were clinically indicated, such as referring her to another therapist or arranging for hospitalization or a different type of treatment, but the therapist would not extend the time for which he or she would personally treat the patient.)

In his later writings (Mann and Goldman 1991), Mann softened this prohibition against further therapeutic contact. The case of Ms. A is a good example. When Ms. A called her therapist 2 months after her last session, saying things were "quite bad," he promptly saw her for two additional sessions, focusing on her difficulties dealing with separation. Ms. A related a dream of how she does things for people and is abandoned nonetheless. The therapist replied that his ending the therapy did not mean that he did not care about her.

Approximately 6 months later, Ms. A called again, this time to say that she was doing well herself but wanted to work on her relationship with her husband. Subsequently, Ms. A and her husband were seen conjointly for four weekly sessions. The need for couple's work was a consequence of Ms. A's dealing more directly with her dissatisfaction with her husband. In the couple's sessions, both came to realize how they inflicted pain on the other rather than directly expressing their respective needs and wishes.

Mann concluded his summary of this difficult case by pointing out its complexities—such as the patient's long history of somatic preoccupations with multiple medical workups. He concluded that Ms. A had made marked gains in TLP, particularly with regard to an increase in functioning (both personally and socially) and self-esteem and a diminishment of her harsh, self-punitive thoughts, although she continued to struggle with her conflicts.

■ EMPIRICAL FINDINGS

Most investigations of the clinical effectiveness of TLP have been based on clinical case reports like that of Ms. A. The empirical outcome studies (Joyce and Piper 1990; Shefler et al. 1995; Witztum et al. 1989) have suggested that for highly selected patients, TLP results in significant therapeutic gains (symptom reduction, improved social functioning, increased self-esteem) that are maintained for up to 2 years after termination. Results from one study (Shefler and Tishby 1998) indicate that interjudge agreement about the central issue is positively correlated with outcome. The results of another study (Joyce and Piper 1990), however, suggest that TLP patients may not encounter a negative transference phase in the middle of treatment, as proposed by the model.

■ RELEVANCE FOR MANAGED CARE

The perspective of managed care is consistent with the 12 sessions of TLP and its philosophical emphasis on making the most of limited time. However, managed care would be at variance with TLP's exploring the patient's central issue, which is thought to underlie the development of symptoms. In addition, the model in managed care today views the therapist as a resource for the patient, who can see him or her for intermittent therapy throughout his or her life, much like the family practitioner. This viewpoint is inconsistent with TLP's more rigid stance regarding the definitive ending of the therapeutic relationship.

Because TLP is best for higher-functioning patients, it may be useful for only a small percentage of people seeking help in a managed care setting. However, this existential approach could be very helpful for healthier patients whose passivity and dependency on the medical care system are manifestations of their inability to separate from caregivers (whether real or longed for). In this regard it seems ideally suited for patients who are symptomatic because of difficulties in dealing with separation.

■ REFERENCES

Joyce A, Piper WE: An examination of Mann's model of time-limited individual psychotherapy. Can J Psychiatry 35:41–49, 1990

Mann J: Time-Limited Psychotherapy. Cambridge, MA, Harvard University Press, 1973

Mann J, Goldman R: A Casebook in Time-Limited Psychotherapy. Northvale, NJ, Jason Aronson, 1991

Shefler G, Tishby O: Interjudge reliability and agreement about the patient's central issue in Time-Limited Psychotherapy (TLP) and its relation to TLP outcome. Psychother Res 8:426–438, 1998

Shefler G, Dasberg H, Ben-Shakhar G: A randomized controlled outcome and follow-up study of Mann's time-limited psychotherapy. J Consult Clin Psychol 63:585–593, 1995

Witztum E, Dasberg H, Shefler G: A two-year follow-up of time limited brief therapy in a community mental health center in Jerusalem. Isr J Psychiatry Relat Sci 26:244–258, 1989

4

INTERPERSONAL PSYCHOTHERAPY FOR PATIENTS WITH DEPRESSION

The assumption underlying interpersonal psychotherapy (IPT) is that clinical symptoms occur in "an interpersonal context and that psychotherapeutic interventions directed at this interpersonal context will facilitate the patient's recovery" (Klerman et al. 1984, pp. 5–6). Although interpersonal difficulties may not be the sine qua non for producing emotional problems, they are strongly intertwined with them. For example, difficulties in interpersonal relations in childhood (e.g., loss of a parent, family discord, abuse) are strongly predictive of adult depression. In turn, adult depression is strongly correlated with further interpersonal difficulties (e.g., emotional dependency, withdrawal, interpersonal friction).

Although IPT was developed as a focused, time-limited treatment (14–18 weekly sessions) for depression, its strategies and principles have been modified for use in dealing with other psychiatric problems (Klerman and Weissman 1993; Weissman et al. 2000). In this chapter, we present the application of IPT for its most common target syndrome—depression. In particular, IPT is especially useful in the treatment of depressed individuals who have medical illnesses. For this chapter's clinical illustration, we consider the topic of IPT with depressed HIV-positive outpatients.

IPT initially evolved from the New Haven–Boston Collaborative Depression Research Project. A book, *Interpersonal Psycho-*

> **Consider this approach for patients who:**
>
> Are given a diagnosis of depression, particularly if they are
> - Going through a role transition (e.g., divorce, retirement, leaving home, illness)
> - Experiencing overt or covert conflicts with a significant other (usually accompanied by feelings that nothing can be done or there are irreconcilable differences)
> - Having abnormal grief reactions (i.e., not progressing through the various phases of the normal mourning process)
> - Evidencing social isolation with or without deficiencies in social skills

therapy of Depression (Klerman et al. 1984), was derived from the training manual and provides a good, practical resource for clinical practitioners who are interested in learning how to implement IPT in their own practices. In this chapter, we highlight the major tenets from that book and present current empirical data and more recent clinical applications. In addition, there is now an IPT guide for patients (Weissman 1995).

■ BASIC PRINCIPLES

Klerman et al. (1984) state that IPT is not a new psychotherapy, because many of its concepts and techniques are part of the standard armamentarium of psychodynamically trained therapists. However, IPT does systematize and operationalize an approach to the treatment of depression. Table 4–1 compares IPT with other, noninterpersonally focused, dynamic therapies. As is seen from Table 4–1, IPT focuses on 1) interpersonal relations (social roles and interactions among people) versus object relations or intrapsychic phenomena, 2) role expectations and disputes versus internal conflicts and wishes, and 3) here-and-now transactions versus childhood or past experiences.

TABLE 4–1. Comparison of interpersonal psychotherapy with other psychotherapies

Interpersonal psychotherapy	Non-interpersonal psychotherapy
What has contributed to this patient's depression right now?	Why did the patient become what he or she is, and/or where is the patient going?
What are the current stresses?	What was the patient's childhood like?
Who are the key persons involved in the current stress? What are the current disputes and disappointments?	What is the patient's character?
Is the patient learning how to cope with the problem?	Is the patient cured?
What are the patient's assets?	What are the patient's defenses?
How can I help the patient ventilate painful emotions—talk about situations that evoke guilt, shame, and resentment?	How can I find out why this patient feels guilty, ashamed, or resentful?
How can I help the patient clarify his or her wishes and have more satisfying relationships with others?	How can I understand the patient's fantasy life and help him or her gain insight into the origins of present behavior?
How can I correct misinformation and suggest alternatives?	How can I help the patient discover false or incorrect ideas?

Source. Reprinted from Klerman GL, Weissman MM, Rounsaville BJ, et al: *Interpersonal Psychotherapy of Depression.* New York, Basic Books, 1984. Copyright 1984 by Gerald L. Klerman, Myrna M. Weissman, Bruce J. Rounsaville, and Eve S. Chevron. Used with permission of Basic Books, a member of Perseus Books, L.L.C.

■ SELECTION CRITERIA

Neither Klerman et al. (1984) nor Weissman et al. (2000) specify selection criteria for IPT for depression. (The entry *Selection* does not appear in the index of either book.) The original treatment was developed for nonpsychotic, nonbipolar, depressed outpatients. The originators of IPT do state that the brief time interval of IPT may not be sufficient for patients for whom depression is severe, there have been many previous episodes, the time between episodes has been short, and the social consequences of relapse are great. A brief section on indications for long-term treatment is included in the patient's guide to IPT (Weissman et al. 2000, p. 125). Research on patient predictors of response to treatment has indicated that, particularly for males, social adjustment, interpersonal sensitivity, and social satisfaction are positively related to the benefits derived from IPT (Sotsky et al. 1991). Markowitz (1999) indicates that recent research has found that personality characteristics and abnormal electroencephalograms may also predict differential outcomes in IPT.

Patients taking antidepressant medication do not need to be excluded from receiving IPT. In fact, data indicate that there may be a synergistic effect between IPT and medication that results in a better outcome than would be expected by simply adding the effectiveness of each treatment independently. (See the section "Empirical Findings" later in this chapter.)

■ GOALS

The two major goals of IPT are 1) improvement of interpersonal functioning and 2) reduction of symptoms (e.g., elimination of early-morning awakening and lack of appetite). The overall aim of IPT is to solve problems within a brief period rather than to devise lifetime solutions. Its emphasis is on restoring the patient to an adequate level of functioning rather than on personality change. In this regard, IPT has much in common with supportive therapies (see Chapter 2); however, it also tends to be more active and ambitious than supportive therapies.

■ STRATEGIES AND PHASES OF TREATMENT

The specific tasks or strategies for IPT are divided into three phases: 1) initial sessions, 2) intermediate phase, and 3) termination phase.

Initial Sessions

In the first couple of sessions of IPT, the diagnosis of depression is assessed through a review of the patient's symptoms. The therapist identifies one or two types of interpersonal problems most related to the patient's current depression by obtaining information about recent changes in the patient's life circumstances, mood, and social functioning. The four primary problem areas most frequently encountered by depressed people are the following:

1. Grief
2. Interpersonal disputes (e.g., with spouse, children, or co-workers)
3. Role transitions (e.g., leaving home, becoming ill, losing a job)
4. Interpersonal deficits (e.g., social isolation, poor social skills)

For some patients, treatment may combine several of these principal problem areas. The therapist providing IPT helps the patient to understand the key types of problems he or she is having and the goals specific to those problems. (See the section "Intermediate Phase," below.) In most cases, the patient and the therapist agree on an appropriate focus for the therapy. For example, the therapist might say,

> It seems from what you have been telling me that you have been [state the current problem or problems clearly; e.g., having trouble in your marriage, arguing with your spouse, afraid of losing your job, uncomfortable in your new apartment, lonely in the city, missing your old friends, etc.]. These problems can certainly be related to your depression. I'd like to meet with you over the next few weeks, as we have been doing, for about an hour each time, to see if we can figure out how you can better cope with the situation. (Klerman et al. 1984, p. 89)

Sometimes the patient and the therapist do not agree on the focus. Patients may be unwilling or unable to acknowledge certain problems or their reactions to them because the issues feel too threatening. For example, a patient may be reluctant to recognize that a spouse of 2 years has significantly different ideas about how they should spend their money (an interpersonal dispute) because of fears that the spouse will leave if the patient asserts personal opinions. When there is disagreement on the focus for treatment, the therapist can 1) postpone goal setting until the patient is more receptive; 2) initially set general goals with the idea of becoming more specific as the therapy proceeds; or 3) go with what the patient thinks is significant, with the hope that once this is dealt with, the more central problem area can be addressed.

In addition to ascertaining the focus of the treatment, the initial phase also includes informing the patient that he or she has an illness because he or she is evidencing the signs and symptoms of the clinical syndrome of depression. This "sick role" legitimizes the patient as needing help and exempts him or her (for a limited time) from certain responsibilities. It makes clear to the patient that depression is a disorder—that the patient is not to blame and that he or she will recover with appropriate treatment. For example, the therapist might say,

> It's OK if you don't feel like entertaining and being social now, while you're feeling so bad. Why don't you explain directly to your husband that for the next month, during this phase of active treatment for your depression, you would rather not invite guests and would like a chance to consider social obligations with him before he commits both of you to them? You are going to be actively engaged in treatment with me now, and over the next month we will be working hard toward your recovery. The expectation is that you will be able to assume your normal life gradually and at the end of 2 months should be quite active. As time goes on and we begin to understand and cope with the problems around your becoming depressed, we have every reason to hope that you will feel even better than before. (Klerman et al. 1984, pp. 84–85)

Table 4–2 lists the major therapeutic tasks for the initial phase of IPT treatment.

TABLE 4–2. **Phase 1 of interpersonal psychotherapy: initial sessions**

A. Dealing with the depression
1. Review depressive symptoms.
2. Give the syndrome a name.
3. Explain depression and the treatment.
4. Give the patient the "sick role."
5. Evaluate the need for medication.

B. Relating depression to interpersonal context
1. Review current and past interpersonal relationships.
2. Determine with the patient:
   a. Nature of interaction with significant persons
   b. Mutual expectations and whether these were fulfilled
   c. Satisfying and unsatisfying aspects of relationships
   d. Changes the patient wants in relationships

C. Identifying major problem areas
1. Determine problem area related to current depression and set treatment goals.
2. Determine what are the relevant relationship factors and what might change them.

D. Explaining interpersonal psychotherapy concepts and contract
1. Outline your understanding of the problem.
2. Agree on which problem area will be the focus.
3. Describe procedures and practical aspects of interpersonal psychotherapy.

Intermediate Phase

After the principal problem area or areas are defined and the treatment contract is agreed on, the intermediate phase of IPT focuses on one of the four principal problem areas. Within each problem area, there is first a general exploration of the problem and then a focus on the patient's expectations and perceptions, followed by a discussion of other options in handling the issues involved and, finally, efforts at new behaviors.

Grief

Grieving a loss is a normal part of human experience and usually does not warrant psychological intervention. When people have a delayed, unresolved, or distorted grief reaction (e.g., no dysphoric mood), however, therapy is usually necessary to help deal with the resulting depressive symptoms. Table 4–3 shows the major IPT goals and strategies that are useful in the treatment of abnormal grief.

TABLE 4–3.   Goals and strategies in the treatment of grief

A. Goals
1. Facilitate the mourning process.
2. Help the patient reestablish interests and relationships to substitute for what has been lost.

B. Strategies
1. Review depressive symptoms.
2. Relate symptom onset to death of significant other.
3. Reconstruct the patient's relationship with the deceased.
4. Describe the sequence and consequences of events just before, during, and after the death.
5. Explore associated feelings (negative as well as positive).
6. Consider possible ways of becoming involved with others.

Source.   Reprinted from Klerman GL, Weissman MM, Rounsaville BJ, et al: *Interpersonal Psychotherapy of Depression.* New York, Basic Books, 1984. Copyright 1984 by Gerald L. Klerman, Myrna M. Weissman, Bruce J. Rounsaville, and Eve S. Chevron. Used with permission of Basic Books, a member of Perseus Books, L.L.C.

Interpersonal Disputes

Klerman et al. (1984) define an interpersonal dispute as "a situation in which the patient and at least one significant other person have nonreciprocal expectations about their relationship" (Klerman et al. 1984, p. 104), resulting in overt or covert interpersonal conflicts. The therapist providing IPT does not have any preconceived notions of how best to settle the conflict but helps guide the patient to discover possibilities for successful resolution. Table 4–4 outlines the goals and strategies available for dealing with role disputes.

Role Transitions

In most social systems, individuals maintain several roles at once (e.g., mother, wife, daughter) and make transitions from one role to another (e.g., single woman to wife to widow). Rapid transitions to new or unfamiliar roles or roles that are experienced as a loss or failure may result in depression. Table 4–5 outlines the IPT goals and strategies that are relevant for helping people cope more effectively with role transitions.

Interpersonal Deficits

Some individuals have inadequate or short-lived relationships because they are deficient in the qualities or skills that facilitate interpersonal connectedness. As a consequence, social isolation is quite common for these people. Individuals with interpersonal deficits are usually lower functioning than are those with the other three problem areas discussed thus far. Progress may be slow, and in a brief treatment, only beginning inroads may result.

Because such patients often have no meaningful present relationships, the IPT work of necessity focuses on past significant relationships, the relationship with the therapist, and evolving, new relationships. For people with problems of this type, the therapist can take a very active, directive, and educative stance—for example, teaching communication skills or role-playing anticipated social situations:

Since you are thinking about attending your high school reunion, why don't we pretend that you are there. What are some possible things you could say when you first see some of your former classmates?

TABLE 4–4. Goals and strategies in the treatment of interpersonal disputes

---

A. Goals

1. Identify dispute.
2. Choose plan of action.
3. Modify expectations of faulty communication to bring about a satisfactory resolution.

B. Strategies

1. Review depressive symptoms.
2. Relate symptoms' onset to overt or covert dispute with significant other with whom patient is currently involved.
3. Determine stage of dispute:
   a. Renegotiation (calm down participants to facilitate resolution)
   b. Impasse (increase disharmony in order to reopen negotiation)
   c. Dissolution (assist mourning)
4. Understand how nonreciprocal role expectations relate to dispute:
   a. What are the issues in the dispute?
   b. What are differences in expectations and values?
   c. What are the options?
   d. What is the likelihood of finding alternatives?
   e. What resources are available to bring about change in the relationship?
5. Are there parallels in other relationships?
   a. What is the patient gaining?
   b. What unspoken assumptions lie behind the patient's behavior?
6. How is the dispute perpetuated?

Source.   Reprinted from Klerman GL, Weissman MM, Rounsaville BJ, et al: *Interpersonal Psychotherapy of Depression.* New York, Basic Books, 1984. Copyright 1984 by Gerald L. Klerman, Myrna M. Weissman, Bruce J. Rounsaville, and Eve S. Chevron. Used with permission of Basic Books, a member of Perseus Books, L.L.C.

TABLE 4–5.	**Goals and strategies in the treatment of role transitions**

A. Goals
1. Help the patient to mourn and accept the loss of the old role.
2. Help the patient to regard the new role as more positive.
3. Restore self-esteem by developing a sense of mastery regarding demands of new roles.

B. Strategies
1. Review depressive symptoms.
2. Relate depressive symptoms to difficulty in coping with some recent life change.
3. Review positive and negative aspects of old and new roles.
4. Explore feelings about what is lost.
5. Explore feelings about the change itself.
6. Explore opportunities in new role.
7. Realistically evaluate what is lost.
8. Encourage appropriate release of affect.
9. Encourage development of social support system and of new skills called for in new role.

Source. Reprinted from Klerman GL, Weissman MM, Rounsaville BJ, et al: *Interpersonal Psychotherapy of Depression.* New York, Basic Books, 1984. Copyright 1984 by Gerald L. Klerman, Myrna M. Weissman, Bruce J. Rounsaville, and Eve S. Chevron. Used with permission of Basic Books, a member of Perseus Books, L.L.C.

Table 4–6 lists goals and therapeutic tasks for the IPT treatment of interpersonal deficit problems.

Termination Phase

In the last phase of IPT treatment, termination should be specifically addressed at least two to four sessions before the contracted end of therapy. This allows time to accomplish the three major tasks of the termination phase:

1. Explicit discussion of the end of treatment
2. Acknowledgment of termination as a time of potential grieving, with the patient being informed that it is common for patients

---

TABLE 4–6.   **Goals and strategies in the treatment of interpersonal deficits**

A.   Goals

  1.   Reduce the patient's social isolation.
  2.   Encourage the formation of new relationships.

B.   Strategies

  1.   Review depressive symptoms.
  2.   Relate depressive symptoms to problems of social isolation or unfulfillment.
  3.   Review past significant relationships, including their negative and positive aspects.
  4.   Explore repetitive patterns in relationships.
  5.   Discuss patient's positive and negative feelings about therapist and seek parallels in other relationships.

Source.   Reprinted from Klerman GL, Weissman MM, Rounsaville BJ, et al: *Interpersonal Psychotherapy of Depression.* New York, Basic Books, 1984. Copyright 1984 by Gerald L. Klerman, Myrna M. Weissman, Bruce J. Rounsaville, and Eve S. Chevron. Used with permission of Basic Books, a member of Perseus Books, L.L.C.

to be sad, angry, or anxious about ending treatment but that these feelings do not forecast a return of the depression

3.   Movement toward the patient's recognition of his or her own competence to deal with problems

  With regard to the last task, the therapist, throughout the sessions, should highlight the patient's successes, draw attention to the supports (e.g., friends, church) that exist outside of therapy, and acknowledge the ways in which the patient is beginning to manage more adequately on his or her own.

  Sometimes patients' anxiety about being on their own causes them to ask for more sessions or even to regress to previously inadequate levels of coping. The therapist providing IPT should not be perturbed or dismayed at this understandable occurrence. (See Chapter 3 on Mann's model for a related view of the termination phase of therapy.) To the patient whose depression has been ameliorated but who is still hesitant about ending therapy, the therapist might say the following:

> Many patients have some uneasiness about ending these sessions if they have found them helpful. We have found that a treatment-free period is usually helpful. Let's see how you are doing over the next 8 weeks before making any decisions about further treatment. You can, of course, call me if you need to and treatment will be arranged. (Klerman et al. 1984, p. 141)

If a patient is still severely symptomatic and has shown no progress during the IPT sessions, then the therapist should consider immediately instituting alternative treatments, such as psychopharmacotherapy, a different type of therapy, or IPT with a different therapist.

■ CLINICAL ILLUSTRATION

As an illustration of IPT formulation and technique, the IPT of depressed HIV-positive outpatients is discussed here. This population was chosen because IPT has much to offer in the treatment of chronically ill or medically compromised individuals who develop depressive symptoms and because of the urgent public health need to treat patients who are infected with HIV. Markowitz et al. (1992) considered the IPT format and four problem areas to be especially relevant for depressed HIV-positive individuals. Specifically, they reasoned that:

- The individual treatment format (as opposed to group therapy) is more appropriate when concerns about confidentiality are salient.
- The possibility of flexibility in scheduling was conducive to a physically ill patient who might have many medical appointments or hospitalizations.
- The engaging, active, and reassuring stance of the therapist in IPT, the treatment's emphasis on opportunities in the here and

now, and its fostering of interpersonal connectedness and activity might counteract the demoralization and passivity that often accompany both depression and medical illness.

In a pilot study, seven overlapping aspects of IPT were found to be especially helpful in resolving the depression of HIV-positive individuals (Markowitz et al. 1992). These seven aspects are discussed in the sections that follow.

Psychoeducation About the Sick Role

In the initial phase of treatment, HIV outpatients were told that they had two medical conditions—depression and HIV infection. They were informed about the symptoms of depression, such as feelings of worthlessness and impairments in sleep and appetite. Many of the patients had attributed these symptoms solely to their HIV status, which served only to increase their depression. Realization that some of their problems were due to a treatable psychiatric condition helped foster hope.

Here-and-Now Framework

IPT's focus on present circumstances helped patients avoid dwelling on "if only" with regard to obsessively blaming themselves for contracting HIV. The therapist emphasized that depression was due to present problems and therefore solutions could be found.

Interpersonal Formulation

Before treatment, patients thought that depression was an unavoidable consequence of their terminal condition. With IPT, they became able to differentiate between normal, sad reactions to bad news and clinical depression. In fact, studies have found that most people with incurable illnesses are not clinically depressed (Cella and Perry 1988). The IPT therapist treating HIV-positive patients may say something like the following:

Your symptoms are part of depression, and that depression is related to what's been happening in your interpersonal situation. [Examples of difficulties in the patient's present situation are described.] Although your situation feels hopeless and untreatable, it isn't. That feeling is a symptom of depression, a highly treatable and common disorder. About 1 in 10 Americans become depressed sometime in their lifetimes; they nearly always get better with treatment. Depression affects and is affected by interpersonal relationships. [At this point, the therapist identifies social withdrawal, losses, and altered relationships in the patient's life.] Interpersonal therapy, a brief treatment based on this connection, has been proven to be as effective as medication or any other treatment for the kind of depression you have. We'll try to focus on the stresses and relationships in your life that may be contributing to depression. (Markowitz et al. 1992, p. 887)

Exploring Options

The depressed HIV-positive patients often had the sense that their lives were already over and that they were waiting to die, although most were physically asymptomatic. IPT challenged their perceptions by reframing their illness as an opportunity to assess their present relationships and make changes to correct problems when possible. At the conclusion of IPT, the patients were buoyed by the realization that there are usually always options.

Problem Areas

Although most of the HIV-positive patients had major issues in three or all four of the IPT problem areas (e.g., complicated bereavement, disputes with partners, job loss, social isolation), the IPT therapists focused on one or, at most, two areas to provide structure and promote progress.

Grief

Four common factors hindered the patients' ability to deal with grieving before treatment: 1) anticipatory mourning of their own death, 2) survivor guilt over outliving others, 3) fear of rejection by others should they learn of their HIV status, and 4) emotional numbing from encountering so many deaths of friends and loved ones. The therapists who provided IPT addressed each of these impediments to resolving grief. For example, they examined the patients' beliefs that family members could not accept them if they knew their HIV status and/or sexual orientation and suggested that they test their expectations with potentially supportive relatives.

Interpersonal Disputes

IPT focused on helping patients with HIV find ways to reconcile differences, obtain alternative sources of support, and end unrewarding relationships. For example, Mr. B, fearing abandonment, was tolerating being taken advantage of financially by his live-in partner. His therapist pointed out that Mr. B seemed more emotionally capable of living alone than he had assumed. The patient proceeded to check out this possibility by having his partner leave for 2 months at a time. Feeling like he had renewed options, Mr. B no longer felt exploited or feared being alone. As a consequence, his depression lifted.

Role Transitions

Although the therapists acknowledged dramatic and difficult role transitions in the patients' lives, they challenged the patients' passivity. The therapists helped patients anticipate how to best deal with physicians, sexual partners, bosses, and others, necessitated by shifting roles (e.g., from being asymptomatic to developing symptoms to having AIDS).

The patients with HIV manifested problems at both ends of the role transition continuum. Some responded to the transition catastrophically. Mr. C, for example, was psychologically incapacitated with his first bout of *Pneumocystis carinii* pneumonia. He thought it "destroyed everything." He withdrew, gave up occupationally, and waited to die. IPT sessions were spent focusing on his remaining options. As a result, Mr. C was able to reconnect with a former lover and to use this partner's emotional support to encourage him to go after a previously avoided but desired career advancement.

Other patients responded to learning that they were HIV positive by minimizing its impact. Mr. D never told anyone about his medical diagnosis, even while taking care of his dying lover. When his lover died, he took no time off work to grieve. He continued with his stressful job as though nothing were the matter. Eventually his denial caused him to become emotionally and physically overtaxed, and he entered IPT to deal with his depression. The IPT therapist focused on pragmatic here-and-now options for dealing with Mr. D's inescapable transition from health to illness. These options, in keeping with the tenets of IPT, focused on interpersonal parameters, such as how to negotiate with his boss to obtain a reduced workload. The patient was able to implement some of these alternatives and to accept responsibility for making his life better.

Interpersonal Deficits

Markowitz et al. (1992) chose not to focus on interpersonal deficits in their IPT with HIV-positive patients, not because some of their patients did not have such deficits, but rather because other types of problems would be easier to treat in brief therapy. For example, Ms. E, a schizoid individual, learned that she was HIV positive during a blood drive at work. When she told her strict Catholic parents that she had probably become infected in high school after her one sexual relationship, they were extremely upset. Their negative reaction exacerbated Ms. E's guilt and depression, and a suicidal gesture caused her to come for treatment.

Ms. E's therapist did not address her social isolation but rather focused on her present role transition and her interpersonal dispute with her parents. With support and direct interventions, Ms. E was able to reconcile with her mother. At the conclusion of therapy, Ms. E resumed her typical schizoid existence but was no longer depressed or suicidal.

Therapist Confidence

One reason for the success of brief therapy with this sample of HIV-positive outpatients was that the systematic framework of IPT gave the therapists confidence. Any therapist could feel overwhelmed and hopeless treating depressed people with a terminal disease. Framing issues as interpersonal problems to be addressed in the present provided an active, focused, and organized way to proceed. It encouraged the therapists' hope and thereby made them more engaged with and available to their patients.

Termination

The HIV-positive patients related their perspectives of time running out and the need to make every second count. IPT's short-term focus paralleled the patients' view of time as a precious, evaporating commodity. The patients' urgency to make the most of whatever time was available and their desire to maximize meaning in their lives facilitated their involvement in the therapy.

■ EMPIRICAL FINDINGS

The efficacy of IPT has been established in a number of empirical studies. Early studies demonstrated the efficacy of IPT in comparison and in conjunction with pharmacotherapy. DiMascio et al. (1979) found that both medication (amitriptyline) alone and IPT alone led to equal overall reduction of symptoms in patients with nonbipolar depression. The effects of both treatments together were even more effective, because the medication improved the vegetative symptoms and the IPT helped with mood, suicidal ideation, work, and interests. A study of depressed outpatients 1 year after treatment (Weissman et al. 1981) with IPT or amitriptyline, alone or in combination, found that almost all patients were functioning rather well. However, those who had received IPT (with or without medication) did better with regard to their social functioning.

In the National Institute of Mental Health (NIMH) Treatment of Depression Collaborative Research Program (Elkin et al. 1989), IPT was compared with cognitive-behavioral therapy, imipramine hydrochloride plus clinical management, and placebo plus clinical management. For the most severely depressed individuals, IPT was less helpful than medication but was of significantly more benefit than placebo. (Cognitive-behavioral therapy was not significantly more effective than placebo.) Additional evidence pointed to the specific effectiveness of IPT. Superior recovery rates were found for subjects receiving IPT (alone) and those receiving medication plus clinical management. In a follow-up study of the NIMH study participants (Shea et al. 1992), however, it was found that patients who had received cognitive-behavioral therapy had lower rates of relapse (defined as major depressive disorder or additional treatment) than did those who had received medication or IPT.

In an open pilot study specifically with depressed HIV-positive individuals (most of whom were homosexual or bisexual men) Markowitz et al. (1992) found that IPT (with an average length of 16 sessions) was successful in resolving the depression of 87% of the sample. In a later study, Markowitz et al. (1995) presented preliminary data from two treatment modalities of a randomized clinical trial (paralleling that of the NIMH Collaborative Research Program). They found that for depressed HIV-positive patients who were not acutely ill, IPT was more successful than supportive psychotherapy in lessening depression. Differences were observable by the middle of treatment (8 weeks) and remained at termination. Patients receiving IPT benefited with increased functioning physically as well as emotionally. Subsequently, Markowitz et al. (1998) found that depressed HIV-positive patients who were randomly assigned to receive IPT and supportive psychotherapy with imipramine showed significantly greater improvement than those assigned to either supportive psychotherapy alone or cognitive behavioral therapy.

A recent guide to IPT provides a comprehensive overview of the adaptations of this approach to the treatment of disorders other than major depression (Weissman et al. 2000). The efficacy of IPT has been demonstrated for the treatment of dysthymia, bulimia, and anxiety disorders. IPT has also been adapted as a group therapy modality (Wilfley et al. 2000). Wilfley et al. (1993) reported significant results for the treatment of bulimia with group IPT. The interested reader can find thorough discussions of these and other adaptations, as well as future directions for IPT, in the guide by Weissman et al. (2000) and in a briefer review by Markowitz (1999).

■ RELEVANCE FOR MANAGED CARE

IPT is quite amenable to the tenets of managed care. The active, directive, and reassuring stance of the therapist and the focus on here-and-now problems and solutions and symptomatology (rather than on personality change or personal growth) in a time-limited treatment are consistent with managed care's philosophy of providing the least intrusive, most cost-effective treatment. Furthermore, given current trends toward manualized and evidence-based interventions, the clearly delineated and straightforward therapeutic approach and solid empirical base of IPT make it particularly appealing to managed care systems. Finally, the goal of IPT to help patients become as active and interactive in their worlds as quickly as possible is compatible with managed care's emphasis on decreasing dependency on health providers. In this regard, the therapist who provides IPT encourages the patient to find supports outside the therapy so that the process of change is facilitated by relevant, real-world (i.e., nonprofessional and therefore less costly) factors.

■ REFERENCES

Cella DF, Perry SW: Depression and physical illness, in Phenomenology of Depressive Illness. Edited by Mann JJ. New York, Human Sciences Press, 1988, pp 220–237

DiMascio A, Weissman MM, Prusoff BA, et al: Differential symptom reduction by drugs and psychotherapy in acute depression. Arch Gen Psychiatry 36:1450–1456, 1979

Elkin I, Shea MT, Watkins JT, et al: National Institute of Mental Health Treatment of Depression Collaborative Research Program: general effectiveness of treatments. Arch Gen Psychiatry 46:971–982, 1989

Klerman GL, Weissman MM (eds): New Applications of Interpersonal Psychotherapy. Washington, DC, American Psychiatric Press, 1993

Klerman GL, Weissman MM, Rounsaville BJ, et al: Interpersonal Psychotherapy of Depression. New York, Basic Books, 1984

Markowitz JC: Developments in interpersonal psychotherapy. Can J Psychiatry 44: 556–561, 1999

Markowitz JC, Klerman GL, Perry SW: Interpersonal psychotherapy of depressed HIV-positive outpatients. Hosp Community Psychiatry 43:885–890, 1992

Markowitz JC, Klerman GL, Clougherty KF, et al: Individual psychotherapies for depressed HIV-positive patients. Am J Psychiatry 152: 1504–1509, 1995

Markowitz JC, Kocsis JH, Fishman B, et al: Treatment of depressive symptoms in human immunodeficiency virus-positive patients. Arch Gen Psychiatry 55: 452–457, 1998

Shea MT, Elkin I, Imber SD, et al: Course of depressive symptoms over follow-up: findings from the National Institute of Mental Health Treatment of Depression Collaborative Research Program. Arch Gen Psychiatry 49:782–787, 1992

Sotsky SM, Glass DR, Shea MT, et al: Patient predictors of response to psychotherapy and pharmacotherapy: findings in the NIMH Treatment of Depression Collaborative Research Program. Am J Psychiatry 8: 997–1008, 1991

Weissman MM: Mastering Depression: A Patient's Guide to Interpersonal Psychotherapy. Albany, NY, Graywind, 1995

Weissman MM, Klerman GL, Prusoff BA, et al: Depressed outpatients: results one year after treatment with drugs and/or interpersonal psychotherapy. Arch Gen Psychiatry 38:51–55, 1981

Weissman MM, Markowitz JC, Klerman GL: Comprehensive Guide to Interpersonal Psychotherapy. New York, Basic Books, 2000

Wilfley DE, Agras WS, Telch CF: Group cognitive behavioral and group interpersonal therapy for the nonpurging bulimic individual: A controlled comparison. J Consult Clin Psych 61:296–305, 1993

Wilfley DE, Mackenzie KR, Ayres VE, et al: Interpersonal Psychotherapy for Group. New York, Basic Books, 2000

5

TIME-LIMITED DYNAMIC PSYCHOTHERAPY

Time-limited dynamic psychotherapy (TLDP) is an interpersonal, time-sensitive approach for patients with chronic, pervasive, dysfunctional ways of relating to others. Its goal is to modify the way in which a person relates to himself or herself and others. The focus is not on the reduction of symptoms per se (although such improvements are expected to occur), but rather on changing ingrained patterns of interpersonal relatedness or personality style.

TLDP makes use of the relationship that develops between the therapist and the patient to kindle fundamental changes in the way a person treats others and himself or herself. Its premises and techniques are broadly applicable regardless of time limits. However, its method of formulating and intervening make it particularly well suited for the so-called difficult patient seen in brief or time-limited therapy.

TLDP embraces an interpersonal perspective, as exemplified by the work of Sullivan (1953) and is consistent with the view of modern interpersonal theorists (e.g., Greenberg and Mitchell 1983). Data from child development research (e.g., Stern 1985) have pointed to how one's world is essentially interpersonal. As such, the search for and maintenance of human relatedness is considered to be a major

Portions of this chapter were reprinted from Levenson H: *Time-Limited Dynamic Psychotherapy: A Guide to Clinical Practice.* New York, Basic Books, 1995. Copyright 1995. Used with permission of Basic Books, a member of Perseus Books, L.L.C.

Consider this approach for patients who:

- Have rigid, self-defeating personality styles (often indicative of personality disorders)
- Have a history of dysfunctional interpersonal relationships
- Are difficult patients who are off-putting to treating professionals
- Exhibit negativism, dependency, disrespect, or externalization
- Become depressed, anxious, or dysfunctional at work or home due to chronic interpersonal difficulties

---

motivating force within all human beings. This relational view is in sharp contrast to that of classical psychoanalysis, which emphasizes predetermined mental structures to deal with conflicts between the gratification of instinctual impulses and societal constraints.

A treatment manual describing TLDP was developed for research purposes and published in book form as *Psychotherapy in a New Key: A Guide to Time-Limited Dynamic Psychotherapy* (Strupp and Binder 1984). In a more recently published clinical casebook, *Time-Limited Dynamic Psychotherapy: A Guide to Clinical Practice*, Levenson (1995) translates the principles and strategies of TLDP into pragmatically useful ways of thinking and intervening for the practitioner. She also places more emphasis on encouraging behavioral changes and promoting experiential learning and less on insight through interpretation. Her most recent conceptualization of TLDP (Levenson, in press) is from an integrationist perspective that incorporates theories and techniques from a wide range of approaches (e.g., experiential, systemic, cognitive-behavioral).

■ CONCEPTUAL FRAMEWORK

Assumptions

The TLDP model makes five basic assumptions, which are described here.

1. **Maladaptive relationship patterns learned in the past.** Disturbances in adult interpersonal relatedness usually stem from faulty relationships with early caregivers, most frequently in the parental home. The child learns that he or she must behave in certain ways in order to stay emotionally connected with others (Bowlby 1973). These learned behaviors form the building blocks of what will become organized and encoded experiential, affective, and cognitive data (interpersonal schemas) informing one about the nature of human relatedness.

2. **Interactive style maintained in the present.** Although one's dysfunctional interactive style is learned early in life, this style must be supported in the person's present adult life for the interpersonal difficulties to continue. The individual's personality is not seen as fixed at a certain point, but rather as continually changing as it interacts with others. Data from neurobiology seem confirmatory, that while relationships play a crucial role in the early years, this "shaping process occurs throughout life" (Siegel 1999, p. 4). For example, if a child has learned to be placating and deferential because he grew up in a home with authoritarian parents, he will unwittingly and inadvertently attempt to maintain this role as an adult by inducing others to act harshly toward him. Thus, dysfunctional interactions, including that of the patient-therapist relationship, tend to be sustained in the present. Accordingly, one can concentrate on the present to alter the patient's dysfunctional interactive style. Focusing in the present allows change to happen more quickly because time is not spent working through childhood conflicts and discovering historical truths.

3. **In vivo reenactment in therapy.** The patient interacts with the therapist in the same dysfunctional way in which he or she interacts with significant others, trying to enlist the therapist in playing a complementary role. From the perspective of interpersonal therapy, this reenactment is an ideal situation because it provides the therapist with the very situation that gets the patient into difficulties in the outside world.

4. **Dyadic quality of the therapeutic relationship.** By entering into the relationship, the therapist becomes a part of the reen-

actment of the dysfunctional interpersonal interaction and becomes a participant observer or an observing participant. The therapist cannot help but react to the patient—that is, the therapist inevitably will be pushed and pulled by the patient's dysfunctional style and will respond accordingly. This transactional type of reciprocity and complementarity (interpersonal countertransference) does not indicate a failure on the part of the therapist, but rather represents his or her "role responsiveness" (Sandler 1976) or "interpersonal empathy" (Strupp and Binder 1984). The therapist inevitably becomes hooked into acting out the corresponding response to the patient's inflexible, maladaptive pattern (Kiesler 1988), or, in terms used by Wachtel (1987), patients induce therapists to act as "accomplices."

5. **Chief problematic relationship pattern.** The emphasis in TLDP is on discerning what is a patient's most pervasive and problematic style of relating (which may need to incorporate several divergent views of self and other). This is not to say that other relationship patterns may not be important, but rather that focusing on the most frequently troublesome type of interaction should have ramifications for other, less central interpersonal schemas and is pragmatically essential when time is of the essence.

Goals

The TLDP therapist seeks to provide a new experience and a new understanding for the patient.

New Experience

The first and major goal in conducting TLDP is for the patient to have a new experience. The term *new* is meant here in the sense of being different and more functional (i.e., healthier) than the customary, maladaptive pattern to which the person has become accustomed. The term *experience* emphasizes the affective-action component of change—behaving differently and having an emotional appreciation of behaving differently. From the perspective of TLDP, behaviors that signify a new manner of interacting (e.g., one that is more flexible and independent), rather than specific, content-based behaviors (e.g., being able to go to a movie alone), are encouraged.

In TLDP, the therapist determines the type of new experiences that are particularly helpful to a particular patient on the basis of the therapist's formulation of the case. (See "Clinical Illustration" later in this chapter.) The therapist identifies what he or she could say or do (within the therapeutic role) that would most likely subvert the patient's maladaptive interactive style. The therapist's behavior gives the patient the opportunity to disconfirm his or her interpersonal schemas. This in vivo learning is a critical component of the practice of TLDP. The patient has the opportunity to actively try out new behaviors in therapy, to see how he or she feels, and to notice how the therapist responds. This information then informs the patient's interpersonal schemas of what can be expected from self and others. In addition, the focus on experiential learning broadens the range of patients who can benefit from TLDP (e.g., patients do not need to be insightful or psychologically minded) and leads to more generalization to the outside world.

New Understanding

In TLDP, the patient's new understanding usually involves an identification and comprehension of his or her dysfunctional patterns. To facilitate a new understanding, the TLDP therapist can point out repetitive patterns that have originated in experiences with past significant others, with present significant others, and in the here and now with the therapist. Therapists' disclosing their own reactions to the patients' behaviors can also be beneficial. Patients begin to recognize how they have similar relationship patterns with different people in their lives, and this new perspective enables them to examine their active role in perpetuating dysfunctional interactions.

The Cyclical Maladaptive Pattern

The TLDP method of formulating a case is through the use of the cyclical maladaptive pattern (CMP) (Strupp and Binder 1984). The

CMP outlines the idiosyncratic vicious circle of maladaptive interactions in which a particular patient engages when he or she relates to others. These cycles or patterns involve inflexible, self-perpetuating behaviors, self-defeating expectations, and negative self-appraisals that lead to dysfunctional and maladaptive interactions with others. The CMP comprises four categories, which are used to organize interpersonal information about the patient. These four categories are shown in Table 5–1.

In addition to these four categories, the therapist should also consider his or her reactions to the patient, asking how he or she feels being in the room with this patient and what he or she is pulled to do or not do. The therapist's internal and external responses to the patient provide important sources of information for understanding the patient's lifelong dysfunctional interactive pattern. One's reactions to the patient should make sense, given the patient's interpersonal pattern.

TABLE 5–1. Cyclical maladaptive pattern categories

1. Acts of the self: Thoughts, feelings, motives, perceptions, and behaviors of the patient of an interpersonal nature. For example, "I think strangers don't want to have anything to do with me" (thought). "I am afraid to take the promotion" (feeling). "I wish I were the life of the party" (motive). "It seemed she was on my side" (perception). "I start crying when I get angry with my husband" (behavior).

2. Expectations of others' reactions: How the patient imagines others will react to him or her in response to some interpersonal behavior (act of the self). "My boss will fire me if I make a mistake." "If I go to the dance, no one will ask me to dance."

3. Acts of others toward the self: Actual behaviors of other people, as observed and interpreted by the patient. "When I made a mistake at work, my boss avoided me." "He asked me to dance, but only because he felt sorry for me."

4. Acts of the self toward the self: Behaviors or attitudes toward oneself by oneself. "When I disappoint someone, I tend to berate myself." "When no one asked me to dance, I told myself it's because I'm fat, ugly, and unlovable."

A successful TLDP formulation should provide a blueprint for the entire therapy; however, it should always be considered as a work in progress that is meant to be refined as the therapy proceeds. The CMP describes the nature of the problem, leads to the delineation of the goals, serves as a guide for interventions, enables the therapist to anticipate reenactments within the context of the therapeutic interaction, and provides a way to assess whether the therapy is on the right track, in terms of both outcome at termination and "mini-outcomes" in sessions. The CMP is not necessarily, but may well be, shared with the patient, depending on the patient's abilities to deal with the material.

■ INCLUSION AND EXCLUSION CRITERIA

Five major selection criteria are used in determining TLDP's appropriateness for a patient. (However, TLDP may be helpful to a patient even when these criteria are not quite met, as long as adequate descriptions of the patient's interpersonal transactions can be elicited [Levenson, in press]).

1. Patients must be in emotional discomfort so that they are motivated to endure the often challenging and painful process of change and to make sacrifices of time, effort, and money as required by therapy.
2. Patients must come for appointments and engage with the therapist, or at least talk. Initially, such an attitude may be fostered by hope or faith in a positive outcome. Later, it might stem from actual experiences of the therapist as a helpful partner.
3. Patients must be willing to consider how their relationships have contributed to distressing symptoms, negative attitudes, and/or behavioral difficulties. Suitable patients do not actually have to walk in the door indicating that they have difficulties in relating to others. Rather, in the give-and-take of the therapeutic encounter, they must evidence signs of being willing to consider the possibility that they have problems relating to others.

4. Patients need to be willing to examine feelings that may hinder more successful relationships and those that may foster more dysfunctional ones.
5. Patients should be capable of having a meaningful relationship with the therapist. The patient must have the capacity to experience and relate to others as separate, whole persons so that new interpersonal experiences can be perceived and reenactments of dysfunctional relationships within the therapy can be examined.

The type of patient for whom TLDP is not suitable is one who is not able to attend to the process of a verbal give-and-take with the therapist (e.g., a patient with delirium, dementia, or psychosis) or who cannot tolerate the active, interpretative, interactive therapy process, which often heightens anxiety (e.g., a patient who has impulse control problems, abuses alcohol or other drugs, or has a history of repeated suicide attempts).

■ TREATMENT

Table 5–2 lists the steps in TLDP intervention. These steps should not be thought of as separate techniques applied in a linear, rigid fashion, but rather as guidelines for the therapist to be used in a fluid and interactive manner.

In the initial sessions, the therapist lets the patient tell his or her own story (step 1) rather than relying on the traditional psychiatric interview. By listening to how the patient tells his or her story (e.g., deferentially, cautiously, dramatically) as well as to the content of the story, the therapist can learn much about the patient's interpersonal style. The therapist then explores the interpersonal context of the patient's symptoms or problems (step 2) to determine when the problems began and what else was going on in the patient's life at that time, especially of an interpersonal nature. By using the four categories of the CMP and his or her own reactions (step 3), the therapist begins to develop a picture of the patient's

TABLE 5–2.   **Steps in time-limited dynamic psychotherapy formulation and intervention**

1. Let the patient tell his or her own story.
2. Explore the interpersonal context of symptoms or problems.
3. Use the categories of the CMP to gather, categorize, and probe for information.
4. Listen for themes in past and present relationships and in the patient's manner of interacting in session.
5. Be aware of reciprocal reactions (countertransferential pushes and pulls).
6. Be vigilant for reenactments of dysfunctional interactions in the therapeutic relationship.
7. Explore the patient's reaction to the evolving relationship with the therapist.
8. Develop a CMP describing the patient's predominant dysfunctional interactions.
9. From the CMP, outline the goals of treatment.
10. Facilitate the experience of adaptive relating with the therapist, consistent with the CMP (goal 1).
11. Help the patient identify and understand the dysfunctional pattern as it occurs in and out of session (goal 2).
12. Help the patient to appreciate the once-adaptive function of the CMP.
13. Revise and refine the CMP throughout therapy.

Note.   CMP = cyclical maladaptive pattern.
Source.   Adapted from Levenson H, Shiang J: "Case formulation in time-limited dynamic psychotherapy." *In Session: Psychotherapy in Practice* 1:19–34, 1995. Copyright 1995, John Wiley & Sons, Inc. Used with permission.

idiosyncratic, interpersonal world, including the patient's views of himself or herself and expectations of others' behavior.

The therapist listens for themes in the emerging material by seeing commonalities in the patient's transactional patterns concerning person, time, and place (step 4). As part of interacting with the patient, the therapist will be pulled into responding in a complementary fashion, recreating a dysfunctional dance with the patient. The therapist examines the patterns of the here-and-now interaction, uses the "expectations of others' reactions" and the "acts of others" components of the CMP, and determines whether they match feelings and behaviors the therapist is having in the interaction. In this manner, the therapist may become aware of his or her countertransferential responses (steps 5 and 6). The therapist can then help the patient explore his or her reactions to the relationship that is forming with the therapist (step 7). By incorporating all the historical and present interactive thematic information, the therapist can develop a narrative description of the patient's idiosyncratic CMP (step 8).

From this formulation, the therapist then discerns the goals for treatment (step 9). The first goal involves determining the nature of the new experience (step 10). The therapist discerns what he or she could say or do (within the therapeutic role) that would most likely subvert or interrupt the cyclical, dynamic nature of the patient's maladaptive interactive style.

In TLDP, the most potent intervention that is capable of providing a new understanding (step 11) is thought to be the examination of the here-and-now interactions between the therapist and the patient. It is chiefly through the therapist's observations about the reenactment of the CMP that takes place in sessions that the patient begins to have an in vivo understanding of his or her behaviors and stimulus value. The therapist can help depathologize (step 12) the patient's current behavior and symptoms by helping him or her to understand their historical development. From the point of view of TLDP, symptoms and dysfunctional behaviors are seen as the individual's attempt to adapt to situations that threaten interpersonal relatedness. For example, in therapy, a passive, anxious client began to understand that as a child he had to be subservient and hypervigilant to avoid beatings. This learning enabled him to view his present interpersonal style from a different perspective and allowed him to have some empathy for his childhood plight.

Finally, step 13 involves the continuous refinement of the CMP throughout therapy. In a brief therapy, the therapist cannot wait to have all the "facts" before formulating the case and intervening. As the therapy proceeds, new content and interactional data become available that might strengthen, modify, or negate the working formulation.

■ CLINICAL ILLUSTRATION

As a way of illustrating how the CMP can be a blueprint for therapy, the first 5 minutes of a first meeting between a therapist and a patient are presented. The patient, Mr. F, is a 74-year-old man who was about to be discharged from an inpatient psychiatry unit. He had been hospitalized for depression and binge drinking and was now being referred for outpatient treatment.

This clinical vignette can be used by the reader to think about what might be this patient's lifelong dysfunctional interpersonal problem—his CMP. It can be helpful for the reader to be aware of his or her reactions to the patient—the interactive countertransference—and to imagine how interacting with this patient would pull or push a therapist to behave. After thinking about all of this, one can consider what the therapeutic goals would be—specifically, what new experience and new understanding would be desirable for the patient to have in the brief therapy. Finally, the reader may imagine how this man's CMP might be reenacted with the therapist during their sessions.

> Therapist: Maybe the best way to get to know you is to have you tell me what brought you into the hospital, what's been going on, and how I can be of help.
>
> Patient [*in a whiny, complaining tone*]: Well, it started in June. We were living in San Carlos, my daughter and I. We have four children. But Susan, the youngest, lived with me the longest. We just got a notice from the landlord one day that he was going to move into our apartment, and we would have to get out and look for another place. So I started looking. We had a cat, too. I started looking all over San Carlos and, ah, down that whole area. My daughter was working down there. And, ah, we just couldn't find a place at all who would take animals. So they decided somebody has to take care of our cat—a relative. But we still couldn't find a two-bedroom apartment for less than $1700 or $1800. It was just terrible. And, ah, I would go out every day. And go through the listings—the real estate listings. And go look. I got exhausted and got depressed and I started to drink a lot. I just couldn't find anything.

Therapist: When was this?

Patient: Well, we got the notice in June that he wanted us out by July. But then…

Therapist: So just last month?

Patient: No, no, no, a year ago.

Therapist: You are talking about a year ago? OK.

Patient: What happened was, I started getting depressed and nervous and exhausted and started drinking. [*Sigh.*] We finally found a place that we could afford, you know, $1700, which was way out in Tilton and it was at the end of a dead-end street—way up on a high place.[*Deep sigh.*] It was very isolated. Anyway, I knew something was wrong—I was really behaving weirdly, so I came over here and they started taking me at the Day Treatment Center. I would come here every day to the Day Treatment Center. That was in October. Anyway, I was taking Librium and a sleeping pill [*pause*], but I was still drinking. And I [*deep sigh*]…so my daughter complained to Betty, the nurse, down there about it, and Betty had me admitted to the Psychiatry Inpatient Unit. And I was there a couple of weeks. And then they convinced me I should go to the Alcohol Inpatient Unit. So I spent a month in there and I quit drinking. Ah, but I was still depressed. So I came back one day for this depression to the admissions and they admitted me again.

Therapist: Back to the Alcohol Inpatient Unit?

Patient: No, to Psychiatry. And I was there through June. Well, that's about it.

The therapist in this case was feeling irritated, frustrated, disconnected, bored, and guilty for not feeling more positively toward this patient. She was put off by his whiny and passive presentation. Using these countertransferential feelings in addition to information the patient had provided about his present and past interactions (from the entire session), she derived the following CMP:

The patient is a very isolated, depressed, and dependent man who expects others to know best what he should do. He waits for them to assume responsibility for his life. Others do step in and direct him, perhaps because they feel sorry for him, or because they get worn down by his whiny passivity, or because they feel guilty for not wanting to do more. However, eventually they get frustrated and irritated by his hapless stance and defeatist attitude; they become angry and/or reject him. Although the patient may initially comply with others' directives and demands, he ends up not feeling helped, but rather rejected, unloved, and worthless. Unable to feel effective and nurtured, he feels helpless and hopeless, leading to his increased drinking, isolation, and depression and thereby completing the cycle.

A diagram of this patient's CMP is shown in Figure 5–1.

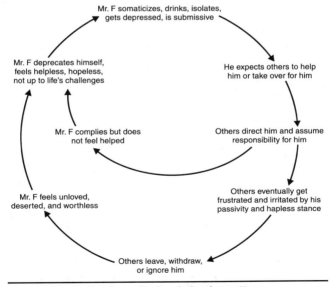

FIGURE 5–1. **Patient's cyclical maladaptive pattern.**

In thinking about what new experiences would help interrupt this maladaptive pattern, the therapist reasoned that if the patient could feel more empowered and more in control of his life—more purposeful, active, and involved—he would be less likely to be so passive and thus less likely to be seen as a whiny complainer by others. The therapist also wanted the patient to have a new understanding that he has capabilities, that he does not need to take a victim stance in life, and that his feelings are important and need not be avoided (by drinking, for example).

An excerpt from the third session illustrates how the TLDP formulation helped the therapist decide how to provide a new experience for the patient. The patient started off by telling the therapist that he had not eaten breakfast that morning.

Patient: I feel pretty low.

Therapist: Do you think it's more than not eating breakfast?

Patient: Well, I don't know.

Therapist: How come you didn't eat breakfast?

Patient: I just hurried over here. I feel nervous.

Therapist: You feel nervous? Why is that?

Patient: I should get some breakfast. I just felt nervous all week, you know. [*Pause.*] I take a stool softener and I had a little accident driving over and I'll have to clean it up, when I get back.

Therapist: Was that upsetting to you?

Patient [*sighing*]: Yes, it was. It happened before.

Therapist: But that isn't why you've been nervous all week.

Patient: My son's mad at me and all that.

Therapist: Why is your son mad at you?

Patient: For not being friendly with his girlfriend.

Therapist: How do you feel when your son gets mad at you?

Patient: I feel very sad, because we used to get along quite well.

Therapist: So you get sad when he gets mad.

Patient: Yeah. [*Silence.*]

Therapist: Is that pretty typical for you, to get sad when anyone gets mad at you, or just your son?

Patient: I get sad when anyone gets mad at me. My kids are mad at me now because I'm not responding to treatment. I'm not doing anything. I'm just sitting around, so I feel pretty sad.

Therapist: What do they mean you're not responding to treatment?

Patient: They tell me I have to help myself, which is true.

Therapist: You're coming here.

Patient [*deep sigh*]: Boy, I feel pretty weak.

Therapist: Do you think it would keep you from talking with me—your feeling weak?

Patient: Yeah. I'm having trouble concentrating.

Therapist: And you think it's just because you missed breakfast?

Patient: Because I'm upset about a lot of things. Everything's going wrong. I'm not doing the dishes or helping to take care of the house, and her cat is mad at me because I chase him out of my room when he goes in and sprays.

Therapist: And that makes you sad, that the cat is mad at you.

Patient [*half-hearted laugh*]: Yeah.

Therapist [*in disbelief*]: And that makes you sad, that the cat....

Patient: Yeah, I really like the cat.

Therapist: You like the cat. [*Yeah.*] So the cat's mad at you, and your reaction is to get sad, because the cat is mad at you.

Patient [*half-hearted laugh; pause*]: There isn't a place in here where I could get a tomato juice or anything?

Therapist: No, not here.

Patient [*distressed*]: Oh, boy.

Therapist: Mr. F, you are saying two different things. You're saying you would have trouble sitting here continuing with our session because you haven't had breakfast; then you say it's more than that. You would have trouble sitting here talking because you're upset about the things that have gone on this week and it would make this session hard anyway.

Patient: Well, they decided to go up to Oregon to visit some people and they just left and I've been alone for 3 days in the house and I haven't been going out.

Therapist: But right here, sitting here now, do you feel talking with me is difficult because we'll be talking about some upsetting things, or do you think sitting here talking with me is difficult because you didn't have breakfast this morning?

Patient: I think it's because I didn't have breakfast.

At this point, the reader might put himself or herself in the role of the therapist and consider what to say or do. A helpful hint is to remember what the goals of the treatment are. When ready, read on to see what the therapist did to try to create a sense of empowerment on the part of the patient—a sense that he could be the master of his own destiny.

> Patient: If I just got something in my stomach I would feel better.
> Therapist: Uh-huh. And what keeps you from getting something in your stomach right now?
> Patient: I'd have to go over to the restaurant, cafeteria over there. [*Points to next building.*]
> Therapist: That's right.
> Patient: [*Sigh.*]
> Therapist: And what would keep you from deciding to do that?
> Patient [*sigh*]: Well, the fact we're having a session, and I don't want to be rude.
> Therapist: So rather than be rude, you'll sit there and be uncomfortable for an hour.
> Patient: Well, I don't know. I guess so. Unless you'd let me go.
> Therapist: Unless I'd let you go?
> Patient [*taken aback*]: Well, I feel obligated to come and see you, because you're helping me.
> Therapist [*pause*]: Mr. F, I'm not sure what you would like to do right now.

The patient was then put in the position of needing to make a decision. The process of interacting with the therapist around the breakfast issue had raised the saliency of his customary way of denying his own needs in favor of what he thinks others want from him. By making a decision (which provided him with an opportunity to take some action), he was able to experience what it was like to take responsibility for his own behavior. Note that the therapist did not interpret or question the patient's claim that he needed food (e.g., as a resistance), but rather gave him the opportunity to do it differently and see what happened. For example, would the therapist become angry at his assertiveness, as his violent alcoholic father did? (The therapist learned this historical information in a later session.)

■ EMPIRICAL FINDINGS

With regard to learning how to do TLDP, research findings are mixed. Although some have found that therapists can be trained in TLDP (Henry et al. 1993a, 1993b), there is some indication that experienced therapists may have an initial decrement in their performance as they grapple with integrating new techniques into their existing therapeutic modes. Bein et al. (2000), upon inspecting the therapies of clinicians after training, found a disappointingly low level of skill in implementing TLDP. Other studies on different (but theoretically related) brief dynamic approaches have similarly found small training effects (e.g., Crits-Christoph et al. 1998). These findings suggest that it is difficult to teach and/or learn to deal with transference and countertransference in the here and now of the brief therapy session. Clearly more work on how best to train dynamic therapists in this modality is warranted.

There is evidence that patients internalize both their own and their therapists' contributions to the therapeutic interaction and that these internalizations are associated with better outcomes (Harrist et al 1994). In a TLDP research project (Levenson and Bein 1993), 71% of patients receiving TLDP for chronic interpersonal problems said they were significantly helped. A long-term follow-up study of these patients indicated that their gains were maintained and slightly bolstered (Bein et al. 1994). Hartmann and Levenson (1995) found that, if therapists can adhere to them, TLDP case formulations convey reliable interpersonal information to clinicians who are otherwise unfamiliar with the case, guide the issues that are discussed in therapy, and lead to better outcomes.

■ RELEVANCE FOR MANAGED CARE

Although TLDP is designed to be completed within the 20-session framework of many managed care plans, its focus on changing personality style (or character structure) may seem at variance with managed care's focus on alleviating symptoms. However, TLDP can be a very worthwhile and efficacious approach for difficult patients who do not seem to improve with more symptomatically focused treatments and whose repeated visits to psychiatric and medical professionals result in large expenditures of time and resources. It is certainly an appropriate choice for patients whose chronic interpersonal difficulties cause them to become depressed, anxious, or dysfunctional at work or home.

■ REFERENCES

Bein E, Levenson H, Overstreet D: Outcome and follow-up data from the VAST project. Paper presented at the annual meeting of the Society for Psychotherapy Research, York, England, June 1994

Bein E, Anderson T, Strupp HH, et al: The effects of training in time-limited dynamic psychotherapy: changes in therapeutic outcome. Psychotherapy Research 10:119–132, 2000

Bowlby J: Attachment and Loss, Vol 2: Separation, Anxiety, and Anger. New York, Basic Books, 1973

Crits-Christoph P, Siqueland L, Chittams J, et al: Training in cognitive, supportive-expressive, and drug counseling therapies for cocaine dependence. J Consult Clin Psychol 66:484–492, 1998

Greenberg JR, Mitchell SA: Object Relations in Psychoanalytic Theory. Cambridge, MA, Harvard University Press, 1983

Harrist RS, Quintana SM, Strupp HH, et al: Internalization of interpersonal process in time-limited dynamic psychotherapy. Psychotherapy 31:49–57, 1994

Hartmann K, Levenson H: Case formulation in TLDP. Paper presented at the annual meeting of the Society for Psychotherapy Research, Vancouver, BC, Canada, June 1995

Henry WP, Schacht TE, Strupp HH, et al: Effects of training in time-limited dynamic psychotherapy: mediators of therapists' responses to training. J Consult Clin Psychol 61:441–447, 1993a

Henry WP, Strupp HH, Butler SF, et al: Effects of training in time-limited dynamic psychotherapy: changes in therapist behavior. J Consult Clin Psychol 61:434–440, 1993b

Kiesler DJ: Therapeutic Metacommunication: Therapist Impact Disclosure as Feedback in Psychotherapy. Palo Alto, CA, Consulting Psychologists Press, 1988

Levenson H: Time-Limited Dynamic Psychotherapy: A Guide to Clinical Practice. New York, Basic Books, 1995

Levenson H: Time-limited dynamic psychotherapy: an integrationist perspective. Journal of Psychotherapy Integration, in press

Levenson H, Bein E: VA short-term psychotherapy research project: outcome. Paper presented at the annual meeting of the Society for Psychotherapy Research, Pittsburgh, PA, August 1993

Levenson H, Shiang J: Case formulation in time-limited dynamic psychotherapy. In Session: Psychotherapy in Practice 1:19–34, 1995

Sandler J: Countertransference and role-responsiveness. International Review of Psychoanalysis 3:43–47, 1976

Siegel DJ: The Developing Mind. New York, Guilford, 1999

Stern D: The Interpersonal World of the Infant. New York, Basic Books, 1985

Strupp HH, Binder JL: Psychotherapy in a New Key. New York, Basic Books, 1984

Sullivan HS: The Interpersonal Theory of Psychiatry. New York, WW Norton, 1953

Wachtel PL: Action and Insight. New York, Guilford, 1987

6

SHORT-TERM DYNAMIC THERAPY FOR PATIENTS WITH POSTTRAUMATIC STRESS DISORDER

Mardi Horowitz and his colleagues at the Center of the Study of Neuroses, University of California, San Francisco, have developed a short-term dynamic psychotherapy for dealing with stress response syndromes (Horowitz 1976). They developed a 12-session therapy to address posttraumatic stress disorder (PTSD), pathological grief, and other disorders precipitated by recent traumas. Their approach has been used with a wide variety of patients and traumatic situations, including bereaved adults, rape survivors, hysterectomy patients, and combat veterans.

■ THEORY OF CHANGE

Horowitz's approach is based on a specific dynamic theory about how people respond to traumatic events. The theory consists of

Portions of this chapter were modified from Levenson H, Hales RE: "Brief Psychodynamically Informed Therapy for Medically Ill Patients," in *Medical-Psychiatric Practice,* 1st Edition, Vol. 2. Edited by Stoudemire A, Fogel BS. Washington, DC, American Psychiatric Press, 1993, pp. 3–37. Copyright 1993, American Psychiatric Press. Used with permission.

Consider this approach for patients who:

- Have fairly recently experienced a traumatic or stressful event (as Gaston [1995] notes, Horowitz generally does not recommend use of this short-term approach for patients with a complex and long series of linked traumatic events)
- Respond to the traumatic event with intense fear, helplessness, or horror
- Respond to the traumatic event with recurrent and intrusive recollections of the event, distressing dreams, acting or feeling as though the trauma were recurring; and show distress and/or physical activity at exposure to external or internal cues that symbolize the trauma
- Respond to the traumatic event with avoidance of stimuli associated with the trauma or numbing of general responsiveness
- Respond to the traumatic event with marked distress in excess of what would be expected from exposure to a stressor
- Respond to the traumatic event with a decrease in social or occupational functioning

three components: 1) states of mind, 2) person schemas theory, and 3) control process theory (Horowitz 1987, 1988). These three components are critical in understanding the impact of a serious life event such as a trauma. After the occurrence of a trauma, a person is thought to evidence different emotional states and patterns than before the event, referred to by Horowitz as "states of mind." A person may develop a stress response syndrome by responding to the event either with denial and numbing (undermodulation) or with intrusive, repetitive thoughts of the event (overmodulation). Indeed, in many cases, the same patient goes through phases, oscillating between intrusion and denial. This phenomenon underlies Horowitz's position that stress response syndromes are phase oriented.

Person schemas theory holds that the meaning of a life event is not initially integrated into the individual's schemas of self, other, and the world. A serious trauma can fundamentally affect the ways in which people view themselves and their relationships to other people and to the world. For example, the avid jogger who has a heart attack finds that his reaction to the trauma is complicated by the fact that he must change his view of himself as fit and healthy and/or his view of the fairness of the world (e.g., thinking, "If I exercise, I am immune to heart attacks").

Control process theory suggests that people use different controls to facilitate or inhibit conscious recognition or communication of conflicts between previous schemas and the new situation brought on by the trauma (Horowitz 1991). Previous ideas about the self and the world before the event (i.e., schemas that reassure one that the world is a safe and predictable place) are incongruent with the fact that a terrible, traumatic event has taken place. People generally experience this incongruence as very intense, negative feeling states, such as distraught feelings, undesirable thoughts, and anxiety. The individual avoids the agony of these experiences by warding them off.

Each individual has characteristic ways of avoiding or inhibiting these distraught states of mind. In the example of the jogger, the man may find that thinking about his heart attack causes such distress that he avoids thinking or talking about the event. Such avoidance can affect his medical recovery, for example, if he were to avoid doctor appointments or to "forget" to take medications.

The therapist must be sensitive to the meaning of the trauma for the individual. How the patient handles the trauma is further influenced by his or her characteristic modes of warding off undesirable emotional content, which is related to the patient's personality style. The goal of treatment for stress response syndromes is to "reduce the need for controls by helping the patient complete the cycle of ideational and emotional responses to a stress event" (Horowitz 1991, p. 170).

■ PATIENT SELECTION

DSM-IV (American Psychiatric Association 1994) defines PTSD as resulting from exposure to a traumatic event in which the person "experienced, witnessed, or was confronted with an event or events that involved actual or threatened death or serious injury, or a threat to the physical integrity of the self or others" and that "the person's response involved intense fear, helplessness, or horror" (pp. 427–428). Individuals who meet these criteria tend to present with symptoms such as persistent reexperiencing of the traumatic event in dreams, intrusive thoughts, and even actively reliving the experience during flashbacks. Other symptoms include distress in the face of internal or external cues that symbolize or resemble the traumatic event and efforts to avoid thoughts, feelings, conversations, people, places, or activities associated with the trauma. Inability to recall the event, feelings of detachment, hypervigilance, and exaggerated startle response may also be present. In addition to these specific symptoms, more generally observed symptoms may be present, such as restricted range of feelings, difficulty sleeping, irritability and outbursts of anger, and difficulty concentrating.

Another diagnostic group to consider is the adjustment disorders. These diagnoses also require some identifiable psychosocial stressor or stressors to which the patient responds with clinically significant emotional or behavioral symptoms. Generally, the diagnosis of adjustment disorder involves something less than a life-or-death traumatic event (e.g., termination of a romantic relationship or loss of a job). However, the clinician should be aware that an individual's reactions to such events may involve pathological responses that are similar to the reactions typically found under more extreme circumstances. The therapy described by Horowitz and his colleagues is, in general, suitable for patients presenting with these symptoms.

More specifically, Horowitz's approach is best suited for patients who have experienced a fairly recent traumatic event. The term *fairly recent* is interpreted very generally: Horowitz's approach has been used with adults who have unsuccessfully grieved a loss that occurred some years previously. Childhood traumas with which the patient still struggles may not be appropriate for the 12-session approach, especially if these involved prolonged, repeated traumatization. Use of this brief approach should also not be used with people who have "excessively conflictual or deficient personality structure" (Horowitz 1991, p. 168). Exclusions include patients with psychosis or borderline personality disorders, patients involved in litigation, and persons who have experienced a complex, long series of linked traumatic events.

Good premorbid functioning, psychological mindedness, tolerance of pain and interpretations, and the ability to quickly form a good relationship with the therapist are standards in the selection criteria for short-term psychotherapy. It is important to remember, however, that patients who have recently experienced a traumatic event may be exceedingly anxious. Intense, acute anxiety can cause therapists to underestimate a patient's ability to engage in a productive therapeutic process. It is perhaps most useful to consider the patient's history of interpersonal relationships, including the presence of adequate parental figures (Gaston 1995). Patients should not have a long history of psychiatric disturbance, a history of antisocial behavior, a psychotic disorder, or less than average intelligence. Acute suicidality may be observed in people who have recently undergone a severe trauma. By itself, suicidality that can be managed on an outpatient basis does not exclude patients.

These criteria reflect Horowitz's work on a brief, generally 12-session therapy format. Patients with PTSD that involves prolonged childhood physical, sexual, or verbal abuse are unfortunately frequent consumers of mental health services. Sometimes these patients present with evidence of dissociation and even multiple personality. Such presentations are generally not considered suitable for a very brief (e.g., 12-session) treatment course. A time-unlimited format should be considered under these circumstances. In addition, specialized supervision is generally warranted in these difficult cases.

■ GOALS OF TREATMENT

The primary aims of treatment after trauma are to restore functioning and eliminate the symptoms associated with PTSD. With therapy, the overwhelming states of distress and avoidance of thoughts and feelings associated with the event, along with symptoms like sleep disturbance and irritability, should diminish. More specifically, however, the patient should be able to diminish the frequency and intensity of both the denial and the intrusive states. Thus, the goal is to achieve a sense of relative mastery over the traumatic event, in which both denial and repetitive reexperiencing are reduced or minimized. One author, Gaston (1995), has further specified the main goals of this treatment, as discussed in the following paragraphs.

Acknowledging and Accepting the Traumatized Self

Many patients who have experienced a trauma or loss are seeking relief from their loss of control over themselves and their lives. However, they may deny that they have been affected psychologically. An initial step is for the therapist to help the patient acknowledge and accept the fact that the self has been traumatized and that the reactions are normal and expected in the wake of such a traumatic experience. Some patients judge their own reactions to a trauma as signs of weakness or poor character. The therapist's calm acceptance of the patient's need to cry, complain, or even feel sorry for himself or herself can help the patient take a more sympathetic view of his or her own reactions.

Regaining Mastery

To recover, the patient must regain a sense of mastery over both external and internal worlds, within realistic limits. An important aspect of the stress response syndrome is a mistrust of one's self and the world after a traumatic experience. Helping the patient to begin to reenter the world, make decisions, seek support, limit external demands, and control the transitions between intrusions and denial states can help counter the feelings of helplessness associated with loss and trauma.

Integrating the Traumatic Information

The patient must learn to accommodate to the new reality brought about by the traumatic event. Irreversible changes, such as death or disability, may have occurred in the patient's life. The therapist must remember that such accommodations include psychological accommodations but also external, practical considerations. For example, a man whose young wife has just died must make arrangements for child care and other adjustments that are directly the result of the traumatic event. The traumatic event, however, also involves psychological adjustments and changes in the way individuals must relate to themselves and others. This kind of goal involves developing new ways of viewing the self, others, and the world so that a sense of the world as an essentially safe place can be restored.

The attainment of this goal usually ensures that the PTSD symptoms will decrease. For some people, however, such integration is extremely difficult. In these cases, it may be important to lower the therapeutic objective to a partial assimilation of the new information into the person's schemas. Developing new skills around specific tasks that have the effect of restoring functioning, within limits, can be very helpful.

Viewing Trauma as a Challenge

The therapist can help the patient learn to view traumatic events as opportunities for growth. Without being Pollyanna-ish, the therapist should hold to the idea of at least the possibility that some good can come of a tragedy and that the patient can move forward and have a worthwhile life. Consider the response of the actor Christopher Reeve to his riding accident, which left him paralyzed below the neck. Among other activities, he has begun to lobby for increasing funds for spinal cord injuries. John Walsh, the father of the murdered child Adam Walsh, responded to his grief by changing how law enforcement agencies respond to child abductions. To fully experience life while recognizing its vulnerability and finality is a high-level psychological achievement. To help patients in this regard, the therapist must be comfortable with issues of life, death, and meaning.

These goals will be achieved to various degrees and in various sequences by different people. In general, the first two goals, acceptance and mastery, are achieved before integration and viewing trauma as a challenge.

■ TECHNIQUES OF THERAPY FOR PATIENTS WITH STRESS RESPONSE SYNDROMES

Intrusion-Denial Phases

A central aim of the therapist in this form of therapy is to be sensitive to the patient's current phase of response. If the patient is in the intrusive phase, efforts to get the patient in touch with his or her feelings may be quite antitherapeutic. For patients who are unable to stop thinking about the event, having nightmares, and feeling flooded with emotion—that is, who are in the intrusive phase—instituting some emotional distance from the event is warranted. This is accomplished with techniques such as providing support, evoking other emotions, and even suppressing emotions. On the other hand, for patients in the denial phase, encouraging feelings is warranted. The overall goal of these techniques is to reduce the amplitude (intensity) and frequency of the intrusion-denial phases and have the patient eventually be able to integrate the meaning of the traumatic event into his or her enduring schemas of life and self. Some of the techniques a therapist can use to deal with the denial-numbing phase and the intrusive-repetitive phase are presented in Table 6–1.

Although mental health professionals are often consulted when a person is in a frightening and overwhelming intrusive phase, sometimes the calmer denial phase is particularly serious when the patient must immediately make important decisions. Dealing with decisions about surgeries or legal matters may be required in the immediate aftermath of a traumatic event. Horowitz (1991) has made practical suggestions for how a therapist might deal with time pressure during the denial phase. Intellectualization can be encouraged in discussing with the patient the pros and cons of particular decisions. The whole process of intrusion and denial may be described for the patient so that he or she can understand the present state of feeling frozen and unable to concentrate or decide. As a last and temporary resort, the clinician may elicit the support of someone whom the patient trusts to help make the decisions.

TABLE 6–1. Classification of techniques for stress response syndrome

Processes	Denial phase	Intrusive phase
Change Controlling processes	Reduce controls: Interpretation of defenses Hypnosis and suggestion Uncovering interpretations	Provide controls: Structure time and events Take over ego functions Reduce external stimuli Rest Permit idealization and dependency
Change Information processing	Encourage abreaction Encourage description: Use images in fantasy Enactments (e.g., role playing)	Remove environmental reminders Differentiate: Reality from fantasy Past self-object images from current ones Suppress thinking (e.g., sedation)
Change Emotional processing	Encourage catharsis Explore emotional aspects Encourage emotional relationships	Support Evoke other emotions Desensitization procedures Relaxation and biofeedback

Source. Reprinted from Levenson H, Hales RE: "Brief Psychodynamically Informed Therapy for Medically Ill Patients," in *Medical-Psychiatric Practice,* 1st Edition, Vol. 2. Edited by Stoudemire A, Fogel BS. Washington, DC, American Psychiatric Press, 1993, p. 29. Copyright 1993, American Psychiatric Press. Used with permission. Originally adapted from Horowitz 1976.

Treating Acutely Ill Patients in the Intrusive Phase of Response

Most of the time, patients seek help for stress response syndromes when they are being overwhelmed with intrusive ideas or emotions. Because of this, Horowitz (1991) is quite explicit about how to deal with this response phase. The reality of the traumatic event usually results in a sense of intense need on the part of the patient, to which the therapist wishes to respond swiftly. For physicians, reactions to this pressure often result in the immediate prescription of anxiolytics or sedatives. Although this is sometimes warranted, it is also possible that it is sufficient for the therapist to be responsive and to establish a treatment program.

The act of talking about the events and having a safe and non-judgmental place to express one's true reactions to it can markedly reduce the patient's sense of being overwhelmed. When insomnia results in fatigue and poorer coping capacities, sedation or antianxiety agents may be prescribed on a night-by-night basis. Smaller doses of anxiolytics prescribed for use during the day, also on a dose-by-dose basis, can be used if the patient's anxiety and distress are preventing adaptive functioning (Horowitz 1991). Given the potential dangerousness of overdose with such agents, the therapist should remain alert to occult suicidal ideation. Horowitz (1991) also warns against the use of antidepressants to relieve immediate sadness and despondent responses to loss. Particularly in the face of a recent trauma, the patient needs to experience and process the natural emotional reactions to traumatic events. These medications are useful, however, if the depressive reaction is pathological and prolonged and meets the necessary diagnostic criteria for major depressive disorder. If psychotherapy alone is not leading to clear, rapid, and progressive improvement, alternative treatments should be considered. However, even if medications are considered appropriate, the working through of the psychological aspects of the traumatic response will be helpful in avoiding relapse once the medications are discontinued.

During the acute phase of therapy with someone who has just experienced a severe trauma, the therapist should be willing to take a very active role. Such work is similar to crisis counseling. More so than in other dynamic therapy approaches, the therapist may directly advise patients to avoid driving, operating machinery, or engaging in tasks for which alertness is essential to safety. Persons already under stress are more likely to have accidents due to lapses in attention, concentration, and sequential planning or because they have startle responses that disrupt motor control (Horowitz 1991). Other points made by Horowitz (1991) for dealing with the acute phase of treatment include the following:

- The patient remains vulnerable to entering a distraught state of mind even weeks after an event. The effects of experiences such as pangs of searing grief, remorse, terror, or diffuse rage are diminished if the person is surrounded by supportive companions. Persons who have undergone similar traumas (e.g., rape) can be especially helpful, and self-help groups are important resources for such patients.
- The more a person has been traumatized, the longer the phases of response will be. After a major loss, considerable accommodation is necessary in daily life and in one's inner schemas. Getting back to a normal pattern of life can take 1–2 years. The therapist should be aware of this and should not push the patient to adjust before he or she is ready. Involvement in productive activities, such as work, are usually helpful in restoring functioning.
- Sleep disruption is a common part of the stress response syndrome. The patient can come to associate relaxation and sleep with feelings of panic and being out of control. This is especially true if the traumatic event happened when the patient felt his or her guard was down. Leaving room lights on, or even having someone sit with the person to watch over him or her while he or she is sleeping, may be helpful in this regard.
- The person who has been traumatized may have cognitive impairments of which he or she is not aware. The effects of alcohol may be stronger than would usually be the case. Tactful discussions of these concerns with patients in an acute state are usually warranted.

- The patient's friends and families often gather right after an event, wanting to know what happened. Paradoxically, the need of the patient to talk is likely to come later, when the family and friends may be getting tired of hearing about the event. It is important for the therapist to be able to listen empathically and nonjudgmentally without trying to short-circuit these conversations.
- Many patients expect to be upset immediately after a traumatic event but are surprised and puzzled, even shamed, by responses that come later. They may fear a return of a sense of losing control or may have doubts about their recovery. Knowledge of the normal phases of grief, including the fact that intrusive symptoms may occur after a prolonged period of denial, can be very helpful to the patient as a way of normalizing what is going on.
- When evaluating the patient in an acute state, it is important for the clinician to inquire specifically about intrusive experiences. Patients may find these difficult to discuss and may worry that they are "going crazy." Here, too, the therapist's communication that these reactions are normal and that more openness about such experiences is helpful rather than harmful can further the therapeutic process.

When the patient does describe the traumatic event, it is important to pay close attention to the details. Sometimes it is important for the therapist and the patient to go over and over the experience and the patient's thoughts and fantasies about the events. It is not unusual for the patient to think that he or she did something that caused the event, which then leads to feelings of intense guilt. One young man was referred to therapy by the court for smashing the windows in several parked cars. This patient reported being distressed about the recent death of his brother in a motorcycle accident. It turned out that the motorcycle was the patient's and that he had known that the bike had a faulty plug in the oil pan. He had neglected to tell his brother of this mechanical problem. He believed the oil plug had dropped out, leaking the oil and causing the engine to seize. The seized engine could have caused the bike to go out of control, thereby causing the accident. For this reason, the patient had tortured himself with guilt over causing his brother's death. During one of several retellings of the accident, the patient mentioned that he had been the one to pull the motorcycle out of the ditch, start it, and drive it home. The therapist pointed out that had the engine seized, he would not have been able to start the bike and drive it. Although the patient knew about engines, his grief prevented him from recognizing the illogic of his own guilt reaction. Once the fact about the engine had been pointed out in the session, the patient was able to let himself off the hook for his brother's death and begin responding to his grief in a more productive manner.

Treating Patients in the Denial Phase of Response

Patients in the denial stage of response, almost by definition, rarely present in overwhelming, acute distress. They may claim to feel down, discouraged, or otherwise dysphoric but do not present with the urgency of patients in the intrusive phase. The danger of this is that unless the therapist is willing to challenge the denial in some way, a collusion between the therapist and the denial can develop. Such collusion threatens to leave the patient with the conclusion that, indeed, the "expert" therapist agrees that nothing is amiss.

To work with patients in the denial phase, it is important to respect the denial, that is, to recognize that the denial is in place for a reason. Someone who has undergone a traumatic event may be terrified of not being in denial. Patients are often quite clear that they see little reason not to be in denial: "Why think about it? Why dwell on what cannot be changed?" Such patients are saying that the only alternative to denial that they can conceive of is an uncomfortable, perhaps uncontrollable, intrusion of feelings.

It is critical for the therapist not to push such patients but to empathize with their need to deny, even explicitly to encourage them to remain on an intellectual level (see "Clinical Illustration" later in this chapter). Horowitz (1991) specifies that a major goal with such patients is to help them "dose" the reexperiencing of the event. They can learn that they can remember for a time and put it out of their mind for a time. Control, rather than total denial, is the goal.

Usually patients in the denial phase will discuss an event but do so in a detached way in the third person, as though it were something that happened to someone else. During such periods, asking for details can help the patient move from an intellectualized stance to a more feeling stance. What exactly did they see? What were they wearing? Did they smell anything or hear any sounds? The therapist, however, should not push, but rather should help the patient to organize and express the experience. The therapist should always be mindful of the degree of safety in the therapeutic relationship so that the patient can move into and out of genuine experiencing and processing of the experience.

Content Themes

Although each person has unique ways of responding to trauma owing to his or her idiosyncratic history, common themes have been identified in numerous clinical case studies (Horowitz 1976). These themes form the basis for the working-through stage of the therapy. Such themes include the following:

- Fear of repetition (real or imagined)
- Shame over helplessness (not being able to stop injury to oneself or to another)
- Rage at the source (including God)
- Guilt or shame over aggressive impulses (e.g., rageful fantasies toward those who have not suffered the trauma)
- Fear of aggressivity (e.g., a woman who lost a leg feared that she would verbally strike out at other women "showing off" their legs)
- Survivor guilt (e.g., an earthquake victim feels guilty for surviving when others in his building died)
- Fear of identification or merger with victims (e.g., a woman became depressed when her home was spared after a wildfire but her neighbors' homes were destroyed)
- Sadness in relation to loss (e.g., bereavement over the loss of family members in an automobile accident)

Cognizance of these themes can help the therapist in listening to patients and helping them to work through such feelings.

Personality Styles

The value of Horowitz's work lies not only in describing the phase-oriented model of treatment, which provides a theoretical framework for directing specific interventions, but also in delineating how such interventions must be modified according to the personality style of the patient. As Horowitz notes, "In brief therapy, the therapist must counter the patient's defensive maneuvers effectively in order to maintain a progressive line of work on the focal problems" (Horowitz et al. 1984, p. 44). The interventions the therapist uses must be attuned to these habitual, defensive modes of relating.

For example, patients with a hysterical personality have a vague and diffuse style that keeps them and others from dealing with important conflicts and issues. Patients with more obsessional personalities, on the other hand, may exhibit a ruminating and detail-oriented style that makes them feel in control. Despite this attention to detail, however, the defensive nature of this mode of relating is apparent in the fact that these patients behave indecisively. Horowitz recommends specific therapeutic counters to the "defects" in these and other personality styles; that is, to lessen the effects of the stress response, the therapist needs to counter the defensiveness inherent in the patient's style. Table 6–2 lists some of these therapeutic maneuvers for hysterical and obsessional styles. (For a more complete description of the various relationship and intervention maneuvers, see *Stress Response Syndromes* [Horowitz 1976] and *Personality Styles and Brief Psychotherapy* [Horowitz et al. 1984].)

■ TRANSFERENCE AND COUNTERTRANSFERENCE

Patients who have experienced severe trauma may evidence unique transference reactions in the therapy situation. Some authors (McCann and Pearlman 1990) have listed a variety of transference

TABLE 6–2. Some "defects" of hysterical and obsessional styles and their counteractants in therapy

Style	"Defect"	Counter
Hysterical	Global perceptions	Ask for details
	Impressionistic	Abreaction
	Limited translation of images	Encourage talk
	Misinterpretations	Clarification
	Avoidance of topic	Support
Obsessive	Detailed perceptions	Ask for overall impressions
	Isolation of ideas	Link emotional to ideational meanings
	Misses emotional meaning	Focus on images
	Shifts meanings	Interpretation of defense
	Endless rumination with no decisions	Interpretation of reasons for no decisions

Source. Reprinted from Levenson H, Hales RE: "Brief Psychodynamically Informed Therapy for Medically Ill Patients," in *Medical-Psychiatric Practice*, 1st Edition, Vol. 2. Edited by Stoudemire A, Fogel BS. Washington, DC, American Psychiatric Press, 1993, p. 32. Copyright 1993. American Psychiatric Press. Used with permission. Originally adapted from Horowitz 1976.

reactions that such patients may have to the therapist. The therapist may be perceived as a potential aggressor, a violator of sacred boundaries, an untrustworthy betrayer, an interrogator or judge, a controller, an indifferent witness, and a potential victim of the patient's aggressive impulses. On the other hand, the therapist may be viewed as a caretaker, a friend, a protector, or someone else who might be as lost as the patient feels. An idealizing transference can take the form of viewing the therapist as the possessor of deeper wisdom about life, as someone who can make sense out of the catastrophe and thereby restore the patient's sense of personal meaning (Gaston 1995).

Countertransference reactions are also varied. Four basic ones include 1) becoming hostile toward the patient, 2) feeling overwhelmed or helpless, 3) becoming indifferent, and 4) attempting to save the patient. The therapist's anger can be directed toward the patient because the therapist fears the intensity of the patient's affects or because the experience of the patient's helplessness challenges the therapist's own notions of unalterable control, invulnerability, and safety. That is, the therapist may become exasperated with the patient for not getting over it because it is threatening to realize some things cannot be gotten over. The therapist may overidentify with the patient as a victim, thereby losing the appropriate distance from the patient's experience. This can lead to the therapist's taking excessive responsibility for the patient and his or her predicament. In other instances, the therapist may become numb to the overwhelming anxiety and helplessness associated with out-of-control, traumatic events.

It should be emphasized that feelings of anger toward a patient's victimizer or other responsible party are normal reactions on the part of the therapist. However, the therapist must at all times be aware of the potential for vicarious traumatization (Gaston 1995) and take steps (e.g., seek supervision) to ensure that the patient's needs and concerns remain at the forefront of the therapeutic endeavor.

■ CLINICAL ILLUSTRATION

Horowitz (1987) describes the case of Ms. G, a young woman who complained of depression because her life was not going well. She wished to examine this problem "conceptually" (Horowitz 1987, p. 79). Her main complaint during intake was that she sensed that she was not reacting normally to the recent death of her brother and to her visit home for the funeral. She was preoccupied with this death and the funeral, which led to associative meanings that she was warding off.

In the seventh session, the therapist explored with the patient the meaning of the death as it related to changes in how she viewed her interpersonal world. To get at this material, the therapist asked her to consciously use her often unconscious defense, avoidance of emotion, and intellectual exploration of ideas (recall her stated goal to examine her problems "conceptually").[1]

> Therapist: But let's be…let's be very rational, very intellectual about it. What does it really mean to you that Sam is dead? [*Pause.*] In terms of you? What does it…
>
> Patient: My life?
>
> Therapist: What does…what meaning does it have? Be very reasonable.
>
> Patient: Well, nothing…in terms of the things like coming in and giving hugs and stuff, it's [*pause*]…it means the occasional letter that isn't there, the admiration that he had for me. That asking for big-sisterly advice kind of thing [*long pause*]. It means I don't like the mention of anything about it [*long pause*]. Um. I don't know, doesn't mean, doesn't mean anything that I can put my finger on.
>
> Therapist: Yeah, you know, we just took that level and it doesn't have any big implications for your life on that level at all.

Rather than argue that it does have meaning, which might raise her defenses, the therapist agrees with the patient that it probably does not. This strategy, of going with the defense, often permits patients to become less defensive.

---

[1]Transcripted material is reprinted from Horowitz 1979, pp. 236–246. Used with permission.

Patient: In a way it does, because it [*pause*]...it really brings home the unreality of things. And, like, he was there on faith. I hadn't seen him for a year, but I knew he was there. I had the faith. I believed he was there. And now he's not there, and I have to take that on faith, too. [*Sniffles.*] I'm so, uh [*pause*], what's real and what isn't? Is anybody else there? Now, all these people that I remember, that I feel close to, that I have faith in [*pause*], maybe they're not real, either.

In the next vignette, from session 10, the therapist and the patient explore the specifics of her recollections of the funeral and her perceptions of her family. This illustrates how the therapist can help an intellectualizing patient verbalize concerns about the emotional meaning of the trauma.

Therapist: Would you go back in your memory to when you went home after Sam's death and you were with the family? Let's go back to that point in time in your memory. See what thoughts you find in your mind then. Relate it to this issue: They're showing you a lot of grief and you're not showing any, and what should you be doing?

Patient: My mother even said to me that she wished I wouldn't go upstairs and read all the time, but at least I could come down and be with friends. But the implication is that [*mumbles something about that she should be with the family, that this is a time to be together*] [*pause*]. And I felt bad about that but also kind of defiant, and, "Mom, this is what I need to do, and I don't have to be running upstairs all the time with a book and some food" [pause]. And, um [pause].

Therapist: What were you running from? You're not running from reactions to Sam's death at that point. I don't believe that [*pause*]. It doesn't hang together well enough. It must be something else, I think.

Patient: You don't think it's because maybe I would have to [*mumbles something about having sad feelings*].

Therapist: Well, maybe. But I don't believe it right now. Let's just...

Patient: That's what I thought that it was. That everything I didn't want to deal with…

Therapist: I think you didn't want to deal with your family.

Patient: Yeah, I think that's very true. [*Long pause*.] I didn't want to have to talk with them. I didn't want to have to be comforted by them [*pause*]. I remember crying one night, a night or two after I came home, getting really mad at my mother and going upstairs and starting to cry out of anger and then using the already crying to try to cry about Sam a little bit and feeling better.

Still later, they discuss her perceptions of crying for her brother.

Therapist: You liked the idea of yourself crying [at the funeral]. You clearly felt guilt that you weren't crying.

Patient: M-hm.

Therapist: Whenever you could cry about something, you'd have liked it to be seen by the people.

Patient: Well [*pause*], definitely I felt it that time, and I was really glad that everybody saw it.

Therapist: You were feeling badly about the way you were, which was angry and disgusted and withdrawn.

Patient: M-hm.

Therapist: And you were also feeling anxious about being sucked in somehow. I mean I think there must have been some anxiety that you would…just fold yourself up in her [her mother's] arms.

Patient [*long pause*]: And I kept being tempted to do that, too. Um, came off the plane with my lip-trembling kind of thing and at various times I could have [*pause*] fallen on her breast with tears and wailed. I am definitely afraid of drama because I know I like it, and it's just that it, it's not…[*trails off*].

Therapist: Well, this isn't the time in your life to go back to your mother's bosom.

Patient: M-hm. But I, I could have just gotten a little amount of approval [*pause*] by breaking down and crying at certain points but I didn't. Or by not being silly.

Therapist: Mm. No, I think you were feeling maybe unconsciously, that that's kind of dangerous, being sucked in.

Patient: Like, I went out of my way not to.

Therapist: You went out of your way, yeah.

Patient: That really makes sense because I can see her just wanting me to stay there, you know, not go back to California.
"Stay here, we need you now."

These vignettes illustrate ways in which the therapist can help
the patient begin to identify and work through the feelings associated with a traumatic event.

■ EMPIRICAL FINDINGS

Horowitz's model of therapy has been tested empirically. One early
study (Horowitz et al. 1981) involved 52 patients with pathological
grief reaction after the death of a family member. Using the 12-session
format, the authors found significant improvement in all symptomatic outcome variables, as well as positive changes in interpersonal
functioning and capacity for intimacy. A randomized clinical trial
(Brom et al. 1989) was conducted for patients with PTSD using
three therapy modalities—Horowitz's approach, trauma desensitization, and hypnotherapy—and a waiting-list control group. Results indicated that after 4 months, treated subjects presented
significantly fewer symptoms related to trauma than did the untreated control group. As is often the case in psychotherapy
research, there were no significant differences among the three
treatment modalities, although trauma desensitization and hypnotherapy had a greater impact on intrusive symptoms, whereas
Horowitz's approach had a stronger influence on avoidance symptoms. These authors pointed out that not all treated patients got better (approximately 60% showed clinical improvement), and they
concluded that some combination of Horowitz's dynamic therapy
and hypnotherapy may be beneficial to traumatized individuals.
They also noted that longer treatments may be more beneficial for
such patients.

■ RELEVANCE FOR MANAGED CARE

Horowitz's time frame of 12 sessions is more in keeping with the limits imposed by managed care than are many other brief versions of dynamic psychotherapy. Some reviewers for managed care companies may be concerned about covering the diagnosis of PTSD. Such a diagnosis can conjure the specter of extremely disturbed individuals who have suffered long-term childhood abuse perhaps requiring years of therapy. This chapter outlines an approach to therapy that is suitable for patients with PTSD in response to a relatively recent and circumscribed traumatic event. As such, it is reasonable that perhaps 12–15 sessions could result in very positive outcomes.

It is important when dealing with managed care reviewers to carefully make the case for the treatment, when appropriate, by outlining how one will specifically target the relevant phasic symptom clusters of intrusion and denial. As with other forms of dynamic therapy in a managed care environment, it is best to deal frankly with limitations of coverage in the therapy sessions, treating such limitations as factors that need to be considered when planning the treatment approach.

■ REFERENCES

American Psychiatric Association: Diagnostic and Statistical Manual of Mental Disorders, 4th Edition. Washington, DC, American Psychiatric Association, 1994

Brom D, Kleber RJ, Defares PB: Brief psychotherapy for post-traumatic stress disorder. J Consult Clin Psychol 57:607–612, 1989

Gaston L: Dynamic therapy for post-traumatic stress disorder, in Dynamic Therapies for Psychiatric Disorders (Axis I). Edited by Barber JP, Crits-Christoph P. New York, Basic Books, 1995, pp 161–192

Horowitz MJ: Stress Response Syndromes. New York, Jason Aronson, 1976

Horowitz MJ: States of Mind: Analysis of Change in Psychotherapy. New York, Plenum, 1979

Horowitz MJ: States of Mind: Configurational Analysis of Individual Psychology, 2nd Edition. New York, Plenum, 1987

Horowitz MJ: Introduction to Psychodynamics: A New Synthesis. New York, Basic Books, 1988

Horowitz MJ: Short-term dynamic therapy of stress response syndromes, in Handbook of Short-Term Dynamic Psychotherapy. Edited by Crits-Christoph P, Barber JP. New York, Basic Books, 1991, pp 166–198

Horowitz MJ, Krupnick J, Kaltreider N, et al: Initial psychological response to parental death. Arch Gen Psychiatry 38:316–323, 1981

Horowitz MJ, Marmar C, Krupnick J, et al: Personality Styles and Brief Psychotherapy. New York, Basic Books, 1984

McCann IL, Pearlman LA: Psychological Trauma and the Adult Survivor: Theory, Therapy, and Transformation. New York, Brunner/Mazel, 1990

BRIEF DYNAMIC PSYCHOTHERAPY FOR PATIENTS WITH SUBSTANCE ABUSE DISORDERS

Substance abuse disorders present some uniquely difficult issues for dynamic therapy in general and brief dynamic therapy in particular. Indeed, most modern brief dynamic therapies specifically exclude patients who are addicted to alcohol or other drugs (Barber and Crits-Christoph 1991; Strupp and Binder 1984). Even very strong

---

Note on terminology: DSM-IV-TR uses the term *substance use disorder* to include both substance abuse and substance dependence. Both abuse and dependence reflect patterns of using a psychoactive substance despite negative consequences. The designation of dependence, in DSM-IV-TR terminology, implies an emphasis on tolerance and withdrawal, symptoms characteristic of opiate drugs but not of other serious drugs, such as cocaine, amphetamines, and hallucinogens. Recently, this emphasis on physical dependence has been called into question as authors increasingly stress behavioral patterns of substance use characterized by overwhelming involvement with the use of a drug, regardless of whether tolerance is present or withdrawal symptoms likely if the drug is discontinued (e.g., Leshner 2001). Distinguishing between abuse to the point of causing problems in a person's life (a given for someone in treatment) and dependence is increasingly controversial. For this reason, many in the field and in the literature simply use the term *substance abuse* to describe the problem of those in substance abuse treatment. In this chapter we have adopted this last convention.

> **Consider this approach for patients who:**
> - Have serious psychopathology in addition to alcohol or drug abuse/dependence
> - Are not acutely in need of detoxification or hospitalization
> - Have a reasonable degree of stability with respect to their addiction (need not be totally abstinent)
> - Do not exhibit signs and symptoms of dementia, other irreversible organic brain syndrome, or other medical condition that can create marked changes in mental status
> - Do not have schizophrenia, another psychotic disorder, or untreated bipolar disorder
> - Wish to engage in psychotherapy (seek self-understanding)

advocates of brief therapy (Budman and Gurman 1988) caution the therapist providing brief therapy to be aware of the possible presence of drug addiction or alcoholism in patients, pointing out the negative effects of substance abuse on brief therapy. Furthermore, psychodynamic psychotherapy and its progenitor, psychoanalysis, have been stereotyped by some authors (Vaillant 1981) as "a waste of time" for alcoholic patients, whereas others have noted beneficial effects of psychotherapy on substance-abusing populations (Dodes 1984; Luborsky et al. 1985). Emerging from this confusing picture are several recent efforts to develop dynamic approaches to treat alcoholism (Levin 1995), drug (especially opiate) abuse (Luborsky et al. 1995), and cocaine abuse (Mark and Faude 1995, 1997). In this chapter, we draw primarily on the work of Mark and Faude (1995, 1997) with persons addicted to cocaine to present some general guidelines for using dynamic therapy with patients with substance abuse disorders.

■ CONCEPTUALIZING SUBSTANCE ABUSE AS A PSYCHIATRIC DISORDER

Substance abuse is a complex disorder that is best conceptualized from a biopsychosocial perspective. This means that there are various known contributors to the disorder, all of which have a real impact on the addiction. The *bio* component refers to the pharmacology of the drug that plays a part in addiction, as do apparent genetic predispositions. The *psycho* component refers to personality factors that are repeatedly observed in substance abusers. These include basic deficits in object relations, chronic interpersonal problems, self-concept deficits, and frequent inability to regulate emotions. The *social* component refers to the complex role that alcohol and other drugs play in our social relations.

The bio component has very recently taken center stage. Addiction has been more or less officially labeled by the National Institute on Drug Abuse as a "brain disease" (Leshner 2001; Wise 2000). This refers to interesting findings that have emerged largely from animal studies and human brain imaging studies showing that the brain chemistry of addicted individuals is changed. Substance abuse to the extent of addiction appears to result in long-lasting brain changes that are responsible for the markedly distorted cognition, judgment, and emotional reactions that characterize addicted persons. Particularly affected are the "motivational control circuits" (Leshner 2001) involving the appetitive motivational functions of the nucleus accumbens, along with discriminative and executive functions of the medial prefrontal cortex, the amygdala, and the hippocampus (Wise 2000). These findings are changing the way in which physical dependence is conceptualized. In the past, only drugs like opiates (morphine, heroin) and alcohol, which result in dramatic withdrawal symptoms, were considered to be physically, as opposed to psychologically, addictive. Drugs like methamphetamines and crack cocaine do not produce severe withdrawal symptoms. Like heroin and alcohol, however, these drugs do result in uncontrollable, compulsive drug craving, seeking, and use in the face of negative health and social consequences. From this perspective, addiction is increasingly seen as a brain disease expressed in the form of compulsive behavior.

This new research has implications for treatment. Probably most notable are medications to address the compulsive craving associated with addiction. For many years, methadone maintenance has helped heroin addicts deal with their cravings, and disulfiram (Antabuse) has been used for alcoholics. New medications are now making the scene. Naltrexone has been approved by the Food and Drug Administration for alcoholism and appears to be quite effective. A new medication for alcoholism, acamprosate, is pending approval by the Food and Drug Administration. For cocaine addiction alone, some 60 drugs are under investigation (DeAngelis 2001). However, despite these bio-based advances, the concept of biopsychosocial is as strong as ever. Even if the compulsive craving is effectively addressed, the social and psychological devastation associated with addiction remains and must be addressed (Leshner 2001).

Environmental/social factors, such as home disruptions, disadvantaged upbringing, or history of parental substance abuse and/or mental illness, have been shown to be strongly related to addiction. Deficits in social skills (e.g., social and work skills), too, have been shown to be important contributors to continuing substance abuse.

Addiction is unlike other psychiatric disorders in significant ways. Probably foremost among these is that addiction involves a primary urge. This urge—the urge to use—can take precedence over relationships, money, food, and shelter. Often what is striking about the addicted person is the compulsive nature of the disorder, that is, the patient's inability to stop using despite the loss of family, job, social standing, license to drive, and other basic factors of life.

It should never be forgotten that, at bottom, the person who is truly addicted wants to use his or her drug or to drink, though without the negative consequences of use. That addiction is often ego syntonic explains why it is fundamentally unlike some other psychiatric disorders. For example, depressed patients do not want to be depressed. Anxious patients desire nothing more than to be rid of their anxiety. Rather than being self-referred to get rid of unwanted symptoms, addicted persons are often in treatment because someone else (a spouse, employer, or judge) has directed them into treatment. In this, substance abuse is similar to some eating disorders and personality disorders.

Within this complexity, psychotherapy can and should play a role. Unlike the approaches to some other problems outlined in this book, the treatment of addiction is much more likely to involve other interventions. These might include family therapy; medication (such as methadone, disulfiram, naltrexone, mood stabilizers, and antidepressants); and Alcoholics Anonymous (AA), Narcotics Anonymous (NA), Cocaine Anonymous (CA), or other support groups. It can be very difficult to treat the severely addicted person with psychotherapy alone (Zweben 1993). This should probably not even be attempted by the novice therapist, who runs the risk of colluding with the patient's wish that his or her problems will somehow go away and he or she will not really need to stop using. Thus, it is important for the psychotherapist to be knowledgeable about and open to other providers and other approaches to the treatment of addiction.

This discussion of the biopsychosocial conceptualization of addiction raises an interesting distinction for the psychotherapist: Is the psychotherapy directed to the substance abuse or dependence directly, or to comorbid psychiatric problems such as depression and anxiety? There is considerable empirical evidence that patients with a primary diagnosis of substance abuse and a comorbid psychiatric diagnosis benefit from psychotherapy, especially with regard to improvement in mental health. The evidence for a direct effect on the drug use itself is much less clear. For instance, there is some evidence of the effectiveness of therapy on drug abuse for persons addicted to opiates maintained on methadone (Luborsky et al. 1985), whereas psychotherapy has yielded much less of an effect on cocaine abuse (Crits-Christoph et al. 1999; Woody et al. 1985).

The approach advocated in this chapter is that dynamic psychotherapy should be considered as part of an overall treatment plan that includes some kind of drug counseling and possibly other interventions as well, such as medications and family therapy. Following Mark and Faude (1995), we believe that, for some patients, it is "useful to understand the phenomenon of drug [or alcohol] addiction, whatever the causes, in the context of a person's life, including an understanding of the person's personality or character structure" (p. 296). For this, dynamic therapy is uniquely suited.

■ PATIENT SELECTION

The selection criteria listed near the beginning of this chapter are presented with the understanding that they are relatively broad. There is little in the literature that definitively indicates which addicted patients respond to psychotherapy. There are data suggesting that a diagnosis of antisocial personality is negatively associated with outcome. However, even this apparently straightforward exclusion can be misleading, because data also suggest that antisocial patients who are depressed tend to respond positively to dynamic psychotherapy (Woody et al. 1985). In general, patients who desire psychotherapy and who seek to understand the self-defeating attitudes and behaviors that have contributed to their current situation are most likely to benefit from dynamic therapy. Patients who struggle with sobriety often wish to discuss issues such as personal insecurities, chronic interpersonal failures, or episodes of childhood or spousal abuse. Such problems are not generally dealt with in Twelve-Step (e.g., AA, NA) or other traditional approaches that focus on sobriety. Finally, as stated in the section "Empirical Findings" later in this chapter, other things being equal, the addicted patient who is in early recovery should be simultaneously involved in a treatment that is focused solely on achieving and maintaining abstinence.

■ THERAPIST'S ATTITUDE TOWARD PATIENTS WITH SUBSTANCE ABUSE DISORDERS

For any therapist who intends to treat patients with substance abuse disorders, a careful self-examination is essential with regard to his or her attitudes toward addicted persons and substance use. The therapist's personal experiences with family members who may use alcohol or other drugs to excess, as well as his or her personal attitudes about drinking and drug use, should be recognized and should not be permitted to interfere with the therapist's reactions to the patient's statements and needs. Most important, perhaps, is for the therapist to see the patient as a *person* who abuses substances, rather than simply as an alcoholic or a drug addict. Viewing the patient as a person with a problem rather than as belonging to a stigmatized category allows the therapist to be more responsive to the entire person and thus able to take a more flexible and understanding approach to the patient. This attitude is arguably the most important therapeutic act and is the foundation for establishing a therapeutic alliance. It has been repeatedly demonstrated that the strongest correlate of positive outcome for persons with substance abuse disorders is the therapeutic alliance (Luborsky et al. 1985; Mark and Faude 1995).

■ TWELVE-STEP PROGRAMS AND GROUP COUNSELING

As mentioned above, the substance-abusing patient in treatment is usually involved in treatments in addition to psychotherapy. Most therapists who work with these patients acknowledge a role for the patient's involvement in self-help or support groups. Any therapist who treats people who abuse substances will certainly meet patients who have had much experience with AA or NA, and thus the therapist should have a working knowledge of Twelve-Step programs. It is advisable for therapists who work with substance-abusing patients to attend a Twelve-Step program. Typically, Twelve-Step programs are open meetings that anyone can attend, and attending one personally is a useful experience.

AA, NA, or group counseling directed toward sobriety provide several indispensable services for addicted patients. Group counseling such as that found in intensive outpatient programs can serve to educate the patient about substances and their effects on the body, the mind, and social interactions; can provide a setting for experiencing hope by seeing other addicted individuals beginning the recovery process; and can help lessen the shame of drug and alcohol addiction by allowing the individual to be supported by others who have had similar experiences. Groups such as AA or NA also offer alternative social activities and friends for people whose previous social contacts may be primarily geared toward drinking or using drugs. Particularly, participation in AA or NA affords the patient the opportunity of help at all hours to avoid engaging in substance abuse or other self-destructive behavior during times of crisis.

To understand patients who are in recovery or are struggling with sobriety, therapists working with this population should be familiar with the Twelve Steps (Table 7–1). These refer to a program for recovery from alcoholism developed by "Dr. Bob" and "Bill W.," the cofounders of AA. The AA approach and the Twelve Steps have been very successful in helping countless addicted persons achieve and maintain sobriety. It must also be stated, however, that there are individuals who respond poorly to some aspects of the Twelve Steps. Statements about personal powerlessness are problematic for some people. Others find the strong references to spirituality in the Twelve Steps difficult to reconcile with their own personal views on such matters. In these cases, a referral to Rational Recovery (Trimpey 1996) or its more recent incarnation, SMART Recovery (1996) may be warranted. Unlike AA, SMART Recovery focuses on empowerment rather than powerlessness, does not rely on a Higher Power concept, does not use the labels *alcoholic* and *addict,* does not encourage people to attend meetings indefinitely (weekly attendance for 1 year is recommended), and has trained cordinators as leaders of the meetings. SMART Recovery relies on a cognitive therapy–based approach that attempts to help the addicted individual recognize and counter the negative thinking that leads to substance use.

It is critical for the dynamic therapist to remember that for most addicted persons, an intense focus on countering the substance use is essential. In some cases, medications (methadone, disulfiram, naltrexone, etc.) may be useful. In many cases, a Twelve-Step group, SMART Recovery, or other specific alcohol/drug counseling is useful to focus exclusively on issues around abstinence, environmental cues that trigger use, craving, relapses, and so forth. The therapist must recognize that addicted patients need more support and more structure for their lives than is available through individual psychotherapy alone.

TABLE 7–1. **The Twelve Steps of Alcoholics Anonymous**

---

1. We admitted we were powerless over alcohol—that our lives had become unmanageable.
2. Came to believe that a Power greater than ourselves could restore us to sanity.
3. Made a decision to turn our will and our lives over to the care of God, *as we understood Him.*
4. Made a searching and fearless moral inventory of ourselves.
5. Admitted to God, to ourselves, and to another human being the exact nature of our wrongs.
6. Were entirely ready to have God remove all these defects of character.
7. Humbly asked Him to remove our shortcomings.
8. Made a list of all persons we had harmed, and became willing to make amends to them all.
9. Made direct amends to such people wherever possible, except when to do so would injure them or others.
10. Continued to take personal inventory, and when we were wrong promptly admitted it.
11. Sought through prayer and meditation to improve our conscious contact with God *as we understood Him*, praying only for knowledge of His will for us and the power to carry that out.
12. Having had a spiritual awakening as the result of these steps, we tried to carry this message to alcoholics, and to practice these principles in all our affairs.

Source. Reprinted with permission of Alcoholics Anonymous World Services, Inc. Permission to reprint the Twelve Steps does not mean that AA has reviewed or approved the contents of this publication, nor that AA agrees with the views expressed herein. AA is a program of recovery from alcoholism only—use of the Twelve Steps in connection with programs and activities that are patterned after AA, but that address other problems, or in any non-AA context, does not imply otherwise.

■ ROLE OF VARIOUS PSYCHOACTIVE SUBSTANCES

Treatment programs and approaches are often differentiated on the basis of the patient's substance of choice. Thus, there are programs for the treatment of alcohol abuse and for other drug abuse. Despite a similar approach, AA is often differentiated from NA on the basis of the kind of individual who attends; for instance, in some places older people with more traditional values tend to participate in AA, whereas younger people with more counterculture values might attend NA. In general, however, addiction is addiction, regardless of the particular substance used. Furthermore, many persons with substance abuse disorders use multiple drugs as well as alcohol. The common denominator is that an individual is experiencing the consequences of abusing a substance and does not seem able to discontinue using. Despite recognition of this basic aspect of addiction, a somewhat artificial distinction persists between alcohol addiction and drug addiction. There are even different branches of the National Institutes of Health that deal with addiction (the National Institute on Alcohol Abuse and Alcoholism [NIAAA] and the National Institute on Drug Abuse [NIDA]). The question for the therapist is, what important differences are there, if any, among addicted persons who primarily abuse different substances?

Our experience is that the primary substance of abuse makes a difference in some treatment decisions but not in others. That is, certain aspects of some abused substances have important implications for treatment. Most notably, perhaps, is that there are medications available for helping patients who are addicted to some substances but not for others. Methadone, for instance, can help a person who is addicted to opiates to control drug cravings, disulfiram provides a person with alcoholism an incentive not to drink, and naltrexone is helpful in controlling excessive drinking. At present, there are no widely accepted medical interventions for cocaine or crack abuse, although a number of compounds are currently being tested (DeAngelis 2001).

Other differences relate to the legality or illegality of the substance being abused. A number of legal substances can produce addiction. Alcohol, for instance, can be used legally by adults age 21 and older. Addiction to legal prescription drugs sometimes involves illegal methods of procuring the drug. However, some patients, typically those with chronic pain, are legally prescribed powerful painkillers to which they have become addicted. Many of these patients are middle-class, older individuals who resist the idea that they are addicted like the stereotypical youthful criminal or junkie. On the other hand, of course, are individuals who abuse illegal substances. Issues facing these patients include the fact that mere possession of such substances is illegal and admission of any use can affect a person's job, standing in the community, or even personal liberty.

Many substance abusers are polydrug abusers; that is, they use different chemicals for different reasons. Some individuals may use cocaine or crack to achieve a stimulant effect and opiates or alcohol to become sedated or to sleep. There is also the phenomenon of cutting down or eliminating one substance, such as a drug, and increasing the use of another, such as alcohol.

For the psychotherapist, the issue is not the substance of abuse but its effects on the individual's social and psychological functioning. Thus, confronting addiction means that the patient must face the social and psychological effects (Mark and Luborsky 1992) of abusing substances, such as the following:

- Grief resulting from lost time, lost opportunities, or lost experiences while high
- Muddled or destroyed relationships
- Areas of incompetence that result from having substituted drugs for solving life's challenges
- Fear of approaching those challenges without drugs or alcohol and without the developed techniques for handling those challenges
- The overconfidence that is often used to compensate for damaged self-esteem

These issues may pertain to any addicted person who has been using for a number of years. Often starting during adolescence or in early adulthood, the addicted person in treatment must face the fact that he or she lags behind nonaddicted peers in developing relationships, careers, and other areas of life. When the addiction develops in later years, the addicted person must face the loss of what was built earlier in life, such as a marriage or a promising career ruined by an addiction. Even without predominant psychopathology, addicted persons in early recovery generally have to begin dealing with such issues, whatever the primary substance of abuse.

■ SUPPORTIVE-EXPRESSIVE THERAPY FOR COCAINE ABUSE

For the purposes of this volume, we have chosen to describe supportive-expressive therapy of cocaine abuse developed by Mark and Faude (1995, 1997) and Mark and Luborsky 1992. This approach is based on the concepts and techniques of supportive-expressive therapy developed by Luborsky (Luborsky 1984). The approach has been set forth in a manual (Mark and Faude 1997; Mark and Luborsky 1992), and its clinical effectiveness for treating cocaine abuse has recently undergone testing in a multisite clinical trial funded by NIDA. As discussed above, it is our contention that this general approach should have relevance in the treatment of anyone whose life has been significantly disrupted by the abuse of psychoactive substances.

Core Conflictual Relationship Theme

For this approach, it is important to have an understanding of Luborsky's (1984) core conflictual relationship theme (CCRT) framework for understanding a person's personality or character structure. Briefly, the CCRT comprises two kinds of responses: the core response from others (RO) and the core response from self (RS). The RO refers to the person's predominant expectations or experiences of others' internal and external reactions to them. The RO could include the other person's actual responses to the patient, the patient's anticipations of others' responses, and the patient's fantasies of others' responses. The RS refers to the patient's own somatic experiences, affects, actions, cognitive style, self-esteem, and self-representations. A third component of the CCRT reflects what the patient desires or yearns for, namely, the patient's "wish." By definition, the wish includes an RS and an RO. These components are usually, though not invariably, interpersonal in nature. Thus, the core RS for Mr. H (whose case is discussed later in this chapter) includes his sense that he is incompetent, foolish interpersonally, and unlikable. His core RO includes the statements "Others don't like me," "Others exploit me," and "Others ridicule me." His core wish is to be loved, admired, and appreciated. Thus, he yearns for others to admire him and to be a grateful audience (wishful RO), whereas his wishful RS is to be the young boy of great promise and talent.

The core RO component for cocaine abusers (and probably for other addicted persons as well) is that they typically expect or experience a range of negative responses from others. These include being criticized, rejected, misunderstood, controlled, and/or humiliated. The core RO component can reflect experiences before or during the substance abuse. In the context of these painful reactions of others, substance abusers may seek solace in a relationship with a drug that seems a more reliable companion and friend than other people. These ROs tend to be associated with the core RS component such as shame, guilt, helplessness, and despair, as well as a sense of victimization that leads to feelings of entitlement, rage, and distrust. The interactions of such ROs and RSs can result in (or result from) great difficulty in identifying, tolerating, and modulating and/or expressing one's emotional experiences. The resulting pain is experienced as overwhelming. In a sense, the drug sometimes serves as a kind of "medication" for dulling the pain of these interactions (or lack of significant interactions) with others.

The wish component for substance abusers sometimes takes the form of the wish to continue using without suffering the consequences. At a deeper level, the substance abuser wishes to have his or her wishes—to be understood, loved, and appreciated—without having to give up the substance. In this way, the addicted person avoids any risk of further pain or disappointment or of having to face the necessary, if not glamorous, responsibilities inherent in a mature, satisfactory life (e.g., taking responsibility for negative self-actions; considering others' needs; responsibly attending to work, school, and daily role activities). Table 7–2 presents some questions for the therapist to keep in mind when interviewing patients because they are useful in organizing the CCRT for an individual patient.

134

TABLE 7–2.   **Questions for organizing a core conflictual relationship theme**

Wish:

What is the patient's central wish? What gives life meaning for this person? What does the patient want from other people?[a]

Core response from others:

What has the patient come to expect from others? Frequently anticipated negative responses include:

"They don't trust me; they don't believe me."

"They don't respect me; they are disgusted by me."

"They treat me in a rigid, authoritarian manner."

Such anticipated responses are often used to justify patients' actions and their response from self. These constitute the patient's *core response from others*.

Core response from self:

How does the patient respond to the frustration of failing to realize his or her basic wishes, and how does he or she act 1) to impede the realization of those basic wishes and 2) to perpetuate the very negative reactions from others he or she has come to anticipate? When these responses fall into a pattern, they are called the patient's *core response from self*.

---

[a]As a patient becomes increasingly dependent on an addictive substance like cocaine, the most basic wishes become increasingly displaced and difficult to recognize. Desires or needs become determined almost entirely by the physiological, psychological, and social effects of the drug.

Source.   Adapted from Luborsky 1984 and Mark and Luborsky 1992.

Treatment Goals

Beginning Phase

The first goal of psychotherapy is to establish what has been called a *collaborative relationship* or *therapeutic alliance* with the addicted patient. However, the therapist should never self-consciously set out to achieve such an alliance. The patient will most certainly experience this as artificial or manipulative. Patients in general, and perhaps those who are addicted in particular, are extraordinarily sensitive to phoniness. Rather, the therapist should focus efforts on 1) instilling a sense of curiosity in the patient regarding his or her psychological functioning, 2) encouraging a sense of hope in the patient, and 3) establishing a sense of purpose and relevance of the therapy sessions early in the therapy.

The first step is to inquire about the patient's goals and central concerns at the beginning of treatment. The patient, however, is liable to come up with goals about which the therapist can do little directly, stating, for example, "I need a job," "I need a place to live away from my mother," or "I need someone to talk to." The therapist must work to frame the patient's goals into terms that can be addressed within psychotherapy. Follow-up questions to concerns such as those just mentioned might be "What keeps you from getting a job?" "What seems to get in the way of finding a place away from your mother?" or "Why is there no one in your life to talk with?" In each of these or similar follow-up questions, the therapist must search for patients' descriptions of problematic interactions with people that can be used to begin developing a CCRT. In this way, goal setting and developing a CCRT become parallel tasks.

In addition to goal setting, the therapist must attend to other issues with patients who abuse substances, including the following:

- Patient attendance at sessions is often poor, sometimes because they are using. The shame experienced by patients after having used can compound the already powerful reluctance to engage in treatment. For this reason, it is unwise for the therapist to adopt the traditional, passive role. The therapist should, in most cases, call the patient after a missed session rather than waiting for the patient to contact the therapist.
- The therapist should avoid being rigid and should not adopt an anonymous, neutral analyst role. The traditional passivity of the dynamic therapist tends to be less effective with persons who have a substance abuse disorder than does adopting a warm flexible, and natural therapeutic attitude.
- When discussing abstinence, the therapist should avoid engaging in arguments or generating an adversarial position by insist-

ing on abstinence. Although the therapist should recommend abstinence from all psychoactive substances, some patients contend that they can control their use or can use another substance (e.g., a person addicted to cocaine might insist that drinking is not a problem). One approach might be to take a "let's see" attitude by proposing an experiment in which the patient is asked to abstain from any drugs for a mutually agreed-on amount of time.

- The therapist should help patients to experience and express how vital they feel drugs are to their lives.

- Finally, the therapist should advise the patient to attend a Twelve-Step meeting. Early in treatment, the goal is to get the patient to try out self-help programs and find a Twelve-Step group with which he or she is comfortable. There are great differences among these groups, and in any reasonably sized town, there should be several regular meetings from which to choose. The therapist should encourage the patient to try several to find one that he or she likes.

Middle Phase

The central goal for the middle phase of treatment is to frame the patient's goals within a CCRT framework and to proceed to work on it. Specifically, the therapist should attempt to tie the components of the substance use into the following content areas:

- The meaning, functions, and consequences of the substance use should be explored. Thus, the therapist should look for how wishes, ROs, and RSs contribute to the patient's incidents of substance abuse. For example, a patient described using after his ex-wife refused to let him see his children. In this example, the therapist explored with the patient his primary wish, anticipation of others' (e.g., ex-wife's) responses, and his response from self (e.g., driving to his contact, purchasing and using the drug, missing work the next day).

- The CCRT is used to illuminate roadblocks encountered during the patient's attempts to become drug free. Even when the patient sincerely wants to stop using, the process is never as simple as "Just say no." For example, a person who denigrates himself and others will have great difficulty in getting help from an AA sponsor, group members, or even the therapist. The therapist should explore how the patient's anticipated responses from others and the response from himself or herself get in the way of achieving the patient's own goal of a drug-free life.

- The patient's difficulties in living without drugs are framed within the CCRT. For example, making new friends, adjusting to a more stable lifestyle, and accepting one's responsibilities will relate to the patient's wishes, ROs, and RSs. Anxieties and resistances to change will become very evident around this issue.

Relapse.   During the middle phase of treatment, careful attention should be paid to any relapse. Drug and alcohol addiction is a chronic, relapsing disorder. Modern theory concerning relapse is that relapses are part of recovery. The fact of the relapse permits examination of the patient's response to it. That is, one can respond well or poorly to a relapse. A poor response is to take the attitude, "Well, I relapsed last night. Now I might as well continue to use, drop out of treatment, etc." A more positive response would be, "I relapsed last night. Now I must discuss what happened with my therapist [counselor, sponsor]. What was I feeling toward others and myself that preceded using?" The CCRT can be used to provide greater understanding of the meaning of the patient's use and to permit expression of the patient's shame, guilt, and tendency to devalue others.

Participation in self-help groups.   The therapist should never become dogmatic about AA, NA, or CA attendance. Some patients never become engaged in a Twelve-Step group but do well with psychotherapy. Others take time to get used to and experience the benefits of Twelve-Step programs. As with other aspects of treatment, the therapist's flexibility about Twelve-Step involvement leaves him or her free to acknowledge that people are different and that what works for one does not necessarily work for others. Nevertheless, for the patient who has chronic problems refraining from drug use, Twelve-Step involvement should be strongly encouraged.

Patients should be reminded that the Twelve-Step program can be available to them long after therapy has ended. Often the CCRT can also be used to examine a particular patient's reluctance to engage in a self-help group. ROs that involve anticipations that people in a group will dislike or reject the patient can be expected to impede the patient's willingness to give the group a try.

Last Phase

It is important to remember that the conclusion of time-limited treatment does not mean the end of the process of recovery. In general, the patient should also be involved in some ongoing therapeutic relationship. Thus, one goal of treatment is for the patient to become invested in a social network that can sustain him or her, help avoid isolation, and provide practical help in minimizing or avoiding a relapse. As with any other dynamic therapy, the therapist can expect to deal with the patient's ambivalence toward ending therapy. Substance abusers may have more difficulty dealing with ambivalence than do many other patients. Addicted patients may experience ambivalence, anxiety, and other uncomfortable states as a reason to use, in an effort to minimize the discomfort. The therapist should not be overly anxious about termination and should help the patient to anticipate and express possible negative feelings associated with continuing the recovery process on his or her own.

Transference and Countertransference

As with any dynamic therapy approach, the role of transference holds a central position in the approach to substance abuse treatment presented here. Also as described in other chapters, the terms *transference* and *countertransference* refer to what is said and done in sessions by the patient and the therapist that has implications and reverberations for the therapeutic relationship and that relates to the patient's central relationship issues. The patient's reactions to the therapist figure prominently in the patient's ROs and RSs as identified in the patient's CCRT.

For example, the patient's reaction to a relatively straightforward action on the part of the therapist, such as recommending attendance at AA or NA, may vary from experiencing the therapist as caring to seeing him or her as rejecting or controlling. If the therapist congratulates the patient on his or her first month of sobriety, the therapist could be perceived as an ally, as condescending, or as irrelevant. Outside of therapy, these types of patient reactions are typically left unsaid and are usually so automatic and seem so self-evident to the patient that he or she does not recognize that these are judgments placed on reality, rather than reality itself.

In the face of these sometimes intense reactions by the patient, the therapist can find himself or herself having reciprocal reactions. If the patient is intimidating, it is natural to feel intimidated. If the patient is acting as though he or she is superior to the therapist, it is natural for the therapist to feel resentful. These countertransference reactions can be used to infer the reactions of others who experience the patient's interpersonal style.[1]

It is important to understand that it is not useful to explore each and every transference manifestation. The therapy session should focus on the patient, his or her current life situation, and how the patient's substance abuse affects his or her life. Nevertheless, it is sometimes quite necessary for the therapist to draw out and make explicit the nature of the patient's transference. According to this model of treatment, transference-countertransference relationship issues should be taken up when such an examination may illuminate concerns outside therapy or when something about the patient-therapist interaction is preventing a meaningful exchange from occurring. Relating this reaction to earlier discussions of the CCRT can be useful for both of these therapeutic situations. If, for instance, the patient's RO anticipates scorn and ridicule from others, this may

---

[1]The therapist's attitudes of disgust or pity toward patients with substance abuse problems, described earlier, also represent a type of countertransference. In this section, we are most interested in the therapist's specific reactions that are essentially elicited from a particular patient's interpersonal style.

underlie her unwillingness to discuss with the therapist a shameful incident when she was intoxicated. This reluctance to trust the therapist may illustrate her difficulty in trusting a new, sober boyfriend who wants to get closer to her. Use of transference interpretations can provide a very useful in vivo experience for the patient but should be used cautiously by novice therapists and should take place under the supervision of an experienced dynamic psychotherapist.

■ CLINICAL ILLUSTRATION

The case described here is that of time-limited (6 months) supportive-expressive treatment for cocaine abuse during which the patient was seen twice weekly (Mark and Luborsky 1992). Mr. H was an unmarried, 26-year-old, lower-level manager at a midsize factory. He owned his own home and permitted a male friend to live there rent free. Mr. H had used a variety of substances recreationally for 10 years, but his cocaine use had increased dramatically in the 2 years before treatment. He reported having felt depressed since high school. Mr. H also reported never having had a girlfriend and never having had sex without paying for it. He insisted that his cocaine use was not a problem and that he would leave treatment if the therapist made it an issue. This latter statement is regularly encountered in such treatments, even though, as with Mr. H, there was ample evidence that his cocaine use resulted in missing work and decreased work motivation. His absences and poor work performance eventually led to suspension from his job and then loss of his house. After a particularly severe binge 2 months into therapy, he was able to acknowledge an overwhelming desire to use cocaine.

Transference Implications

The case summary reveals how quickly the transference can become manifest in the therapeutic relationship. Mr. H implied that his staying in treatment was somehow the therapist's responsibility by his initial insistence that cocaine was not a problem and that any effort on the therapist's part to address this issue would result in his fleeing therapy. Immediately in the first session, the therapist felt controlled and threatened. The therapist chose not to respond from this countertransference, which might have resulted in an argument with the patient. Rather, exploration of the patient's interactions with others revealed a pattern in which the patient tended to get what he wanted from others (understanding, pity) by insisting on setting the conditions of the interactions. His tendency to respond by exploding and fleeing whenever he encountered difficult or un-comfortable situations typically resulted in making matters worse rather than better. By patiently exploring such reactions, the thera-pist was able to get the patient to acknowledge these patterns and their negative effects on his life.

Mr. H's Core Conflictual Relationship Theme

Mr. H's central wish was an intense desire for closeness, love, and affection, but he had no idea of how to build such relationships. His central RS, in addition to using cocaine and being depressed, was a self-image of being a fool, interpersonally incompetent, and unlik-able. His central affective states were shame and humiliation. In light of this negative self-evaluation, his only recourse for achiev-ing his wish (love, affection) was to buy friendship with drugs, money, or gifts (i.e., buying drugs for groups of "friends" or having his male friend live in his home rent free). Not surprisingly, he often ended up feeling exploited and would feel humiliated, explode, and flee the relationship. One method of fleeing the scene was to get high. The central negative RO was that he would be exploited. Con-sider how the CCRT and transference are played out in the follow-ing vignette.[2]

Mr. H, who pays at the end of each session, wrote out a check larger than the agreed-on fee. The therapist put the check aside without observing the amount until later. The next session began:

---

[2]Excerpted from Mark and Luborsky 1992. Used with permission.

Therapist: I noticed you wrote out a check for [amount of check]
    last time we met.

Patient: I thought you deserved it. It was an important session to me.

Therapist: Yes, and I'm glad that it was. But still, is it a question
    that you would pay me extra for it?

Patient: I don't know; I wanted you to have it.

Therapist: You know, doesn't this seem like when you buy Lisa
    and Ruth dinner or Stephanie flowers? As with them, you
    want to let me know you appreciated something, that
    something happened in here that was important to you, but
    it gets expressed in the medium of money, with a gift.

Patient: And then I feel taken advantage of.

In this vignette, the wish to get close to someone, to have some
affection and appreciation pass between him and another person, is
expressed obliquely. Rather than having his wish satisfied, he typically ends up feeling exploited, a pattern transferred from one situation to another.

Noted in Mr. H's CCRT was his tendency to use threats to control people and, when faced with difficult, uncomfortable situations,
to flee from, avoid, or deny the difficulty. Indeed, after an explosive
altercation with friends, he disappeared for a week, flying to another
city without telling anyone. In the course of therapy he had threatened
suicide during anxiety-provoking moments. During one session, after
he had lost his job, the therapist asked when Mr. H intended to attempt a return to work—he had been drug free for 3 months but had
made no attempt to return to work. Mr. H began the next session by
saying that it was time to terminate therapy. The therapist was aware
of Mr. H's lifelong tendency to threaten extreme behavior when
things did not go how he wanted them to or when others disappointed him. The therapist's understanding of the anxiety and distress brought about by the therapist's introduction of the topic of
work permitted him to empathically stay with the patient. When Mr.
H threatened to terminate the therapy, the therapist responded:

Therapist: Can you recall what we talked about last time?

Patient: No.

This did not surprise the therapist. It simply reflected Mr. H's tendency to avoid troubling topics. As the therapist reminded the patient of the discussion about work, the dialogue continued:

> Patient: This talk about work is going nowhere. I don't really care about work. Let's just leave it at that.
> Therapist: You want to drop the topic?
> Patient: I would be more depressed if I worked.
> Therapist: Could you say more about that?

By saying that he feared depression if he worked, Mr. H gave the therapist the opportunity to explore the meaning of his need to threaten to leave therapy. Later, when Mr. H said he "dreaded" work, the therapist asked:

> Therapist: Should we try and understand what this fear is about? Is there another way, other than dropping the matter altogether?
> Patient: I've never done that before.
> Therapist: Well, let's see if we can get hold of it. Tell me more about your dread about this situation, of returning to work.

At this point, the patient and the therapist began a meaningful discussion of Mr. H's relationships at work. In particular, he was afraid of returning to work where he had been discharged because of poor performance while using cocaine at work.

At termination of therapy, Mr. H had been drug free for about 4 months and had begun to work. He had connected with a sponsor and was regularly attending NA meetings. He reported being less explosive with others. Mr. H had not yet been able to form a meaningful relationship with a woman. He was able to acknowledge, however, that his chances for improvement in this area were better while he stayed sober.

■ EMPIRICAL FINDINGS

As previously noted, the manualized form of supportive-expressive therapy for cocaine abuse (Mark and Faude 1995, 1997; Mark and Luborsky 1992) has recently undergone a rigorous clinical trial

(Crits-Christoph et al. 1997, 1999). The effectiveness of supportive-expressive therapy was compared with two other psychosocial treatments, a version of cognitive therapy modified for cocaine addiction and a manualized version of individual, Twelve-Step–based drug counseling. Patients in each condition, including the drug counseling, were expected to simultaneously participate in group drug counseling. Patients in all conditions improved significantly on cocaine use measures, but patients in the individual drug counseling condition improved significantly more than patients in either of the psychotherapy conditions. Furthermore, contrary to the authors' hypothesis, neither of the psychotherapies showed differential effectiveness on measures of psychiatric symptoms over the drug counseling condition. Interestingly, despite the outcome difference in favor of drug counseling, patients were much more likely to remain in treatment in the psychotherapy conditions.

These findings are somewhat puzzling, given previous evidence that psychotherapy, including Luborsky's supportive-expressive therapy, is more effective than drug counseling in the treatment of opiate addiction (Luborsky et al. 1995) and is particularly effective in the treatment of psychiatric dysfunction in addicted patients. Several points regarding the cocaine study should be highlighted. First, cocaine use among patients receiving supportive-expressive therapy and those receiving cognitive therapy significantly decreased. Second, like the therapists in this study, the drug counselors underwent an extraordinary selection process, so they were perhaps more competent than drug counselors found in typical treatment settings. Third, the drug counselors in this study had extensive experience in treating persons with substance abuse disorders, whereas many of the psychotherapists in the study had limited experience with this population (although they were highly experienced therapists). Finally, the apparent lack of differential effectiveness of the psychotherapies on psychiatric symptoms may have been due to the exclusion of patients with severe mental illness. The low levels of psychiatric symptoms prevented a test of whether individuals with serious psychopathology would have benefited more from the psychotherapies.

What can we make of these findings regarding brief dynamic therapy for addiction? A fundamental point to be drawn is that dynamic psychotherapy (brief or otherwise) is an unlikely first choice when the presenting complaint is compulsive, out-of-control substance use. Recall the study by Luborsky et al. (1995) with opiate addicts in which psychotherapy was shown to facilitate outcome over drug counseling. In that study, the patients were maintained on methadone, which may have permitted them to more fully participate in the self-reflection required of psychotherapy patients. Furthermore, the patients in Luborsky's study were, as a group, more psychiatrically impaired than were those in the cocaine study. Taken together, these results suggest that psychotherapy may be most suitable for addicted patients who are both psychiatrically impaired and stabilized. Such stabilization may be achieved by high-quality drug counseling that focuses solely on abstinence. Alternatively, perhaps such stabilization might be facilitated by medications, such as methadone (or some analogous medication for non-opiate drugs). To this end, the first large-scale examination of combined pharmacologic and behavioral treatments for alcoholism has recently been launched (Carpenter 2001). In the future, the combined use of medications and psychotherapy may become the norm for patients addicted to most drugs, much as serious depression is often treated with a combination of antidepressant medication and psychotherapy. But, as with depression, there will always be patients who reject medication or for whom medication is otherwise not warranted. In these instances, psychotherapy will continue to be an important option for patients with addiction.

■ RELEVANCE FOR MANAGED CARE

Supportive-expressive therapy with substance-abusing patients has been tested in clinical trials on opiate-addicted patients and cocaine-addicted patients. These treatments, although time limited, prescribe more sessions than are often covered under managed care plans. The manualized supportive-expressive therapy used in the NIDA Collaborative Cocaine Treatment Study (Crits-Christoph et al. 1999), for instance, extended over 6 months of treatment, during which sessions were held twice a week for the first 3 months for a total of about 36 sessions. The clinical trials testing supportive-expressive therapy for opiate dependence provided 6 months of weekly treatment, or about 24 sessions (Luborsky et al. 1995). Both treatment protocols are higher than the availability of 20 sessions a year that is typically available through health maintenance organizations.

Therapists should also be aware that some managed care companies carve out substance abuse from mental health coverage. In some instances, substance abuse is covered only for medical detoxification, so only patients with a mental health diagnosis, such as anxiety or depression, will be covered for treatment. Such arbitrary and (from a treatment perspective) irrational demarcations between mental health and substance abuse problems can clearly have an impact on the amount of treatment available to an individual patient.

It is our opinion that, despite these frustrating restrictions, therapists should not be dissuaded by limitations on coverage for therapy. With the promise of some newly developed medications, it may be possible to do quite a lot in 20 sessions, and perhaps in fewer sessions. With severe restrictions on sessions, it may be wise to use more sessions early, when sobriety is less stable and the therapeutic alliance needs to be established. Spreading sessions out during the later middle and the last stages of treatment, especially if the patient's life is going better, gives the patient time to experience his or her sobriety and to bring in problems to discuss with the therapist. Session restrictions also mean that the therapist must be sure to work with the patient on availing himself or herself of self-help and other community programs.

■ REFERENCES

Barber JP, Crits-Christoph P: Comparison of the brief dynamic therapies, in Handbook of Short-Term Dynamic Psychotherapy. Edited by Crits-Christoph P, Barber JP. New York, Basic Books, 1991, pp 323–352

Budman SH, Gurman AS: Theory and Practice of Brief Therapy. New York, Guilford, 1988

Carpenter S: Mixing medication and psychosocial therapy for alcoholism. Monitor on Psychology 32:36–37, 2001

Crits-Christoph P, Siqueland L, Blaine J, et al: The National Institute on Drug Abuse Collaborative Cocaine Treatment Study: rationale and methods. Arch Gen Psychiatry 54:721–726, 1997

Crits-Christoph P, Siqueland L, Blaine J, et al: Psychosocial treatments for cocaine dependence: National Institute on Drug Abuse Collaborative Cocaine Treatment Study. Arch Gen Psychiatry 57:493–502, 1999

DeAngelis T: Today's tried-and-true treatments. Monitor on Psychology 32:48–50, 2001

Dodes LM: Abstinence from alcohol in long-term individual psychotherapy with alcoholics. Am J Psychother 38:248–256, 1984

Leshner AI: Addiction is a brain disease. Issues Sci Technol 17:75–80, 2001

Levin JD: Psychodynamic treatment of alcohol abuse, in Dynamic Therapies for Psychiatric Disorders: Axis I. Edited by Barber JP, Crits-Christoph P. New York, Basic Books, 1995, pp 193–229

Luborsky L: Principles of Psychoanalytic Psychotherapy: A Manual for Supportive Expressive Treatment. New York, Basic Books, 1984

Luborsky L, McLellan AT, Woody GE, et al: Therapist success and its determinants. Arch Gen Psychiatry 42:602–611, 1985

Luborsky L, Woody GE, Hole AV, et al: Supportive-expressive dynamic therapy for treatment of opiate drug dependence, in Dynamic Therapies for Psychiatric Disorders: Axis I. Edited by Barber JP, Crits-Christoph P. New York, Basic Books, 1995, pp 131–160

Mark D, Faude J: Supportive-expressive therapy of cocaine abuse, in Dynamic Therapies for Psychiatric Disorders: Axis I. Edited by Barber JP, Crits-Christoph P. New York, Basic Books, 1995, pp 294–331

Mark D, Faude J: Psychotherapy of Cocaine Addiction: Entering the Interpersonal World of the Cocaine Addict. Northvale, NJ, Jason Aronson, 1997

Mark D, Luborsky L: A Manual for the Use of Supportive-Expressive Therapy in the Treatment of Cocaine Abuse. Unpublished manual, Department of Psychiatry, Hospital of the University of Pennsylvania, Philadelphia, Pennsylvania, March 1992

SMART Recovery: SMART Recovery Member's Manual. Beachwood, OH: SMART Recovery Self-Help Network, 1996

Strupp HH, Binder JL: Psychotherapy in a New Key. New York, Basic Books, 1984

Trimpey J: Rational Recovery: The New Cure for Substance Addiction. New York, Pocket Books, 1996

Vaillant GE: Dangers of psychotherapy in the treatment of alcoholism, in Dynamic Approaches to the Understanding and Treatment of Alcoholism. Edited by Bean MH, Zinberg NE. New York, Free Press, 1981, pp 36–54

Wise, RA: Addiction becomes a brain disease. Neuron 26:27–33, 2000

Woody GE, McLellan AT, Luborsky L, et al: Sociopathy and psychotherapy outcome. Arch Gen Psychiatry 40:1081–1086, 1985

Zweben J: Recovery-oriented psychotherapy: a model for addiction treatment. Psychotherapy 30:259–268, 1993

TIME-LIMITED
GROUP THERAPY

The practice of providing therapeutic services in a group dates back
at least as far as the early 1900s (Marsh 190 9; Pratt 1905), but the
last two decades have shown a marked increase in the study of
groups and the use of group therapies (Scheidlinger 2000). This
progression, combined with a growing body of evidence supporting
the efficacy of group treatments, has led some to suggest that
a group therapy program is an essential component of any comprehensive mental health care delivery system, and time-limited
groups have a special role to play within that program (MacKenzie
2000; Steenbarger and Budman 1996). Whereas individual psychotherapy makes use of the relationship between the patient and the
trained professional therapist, group therapies make use of not only
this relationship but also the powerful forces of patient-patient interactions. In addition to the various techniques and interventions
applied by the group therapist, the group itself is, therefore, a therapeutic agent. It is precisely this quality that sets this treatment modality apart from all others.

Traditionally, effective group therapy has been thought of as
necessarily long-term treatment. Changes in the health care delivery system due to concerns over cost containment demanded the development of efficient and cost-effective treatment modalities.
Following the lead of time-effective individual treatments, time-
limited group therapies have blossomed over the past two decades,
and there is a growing body of empirical evidence to support their
efficacy (Piper and Joyce 1996). Historically, the majority of group

Consider this approach for patients who:

Present with interpersonal difficulties, deficits, or conflicts as their
major area of disturbance

Are socially isolated, shy, or inhibited

Feel their problems and concerns are unique and different from
everyone else's

Feel developmentally "out of sync"

Are interested in and capable of the interpersonal sharing involved
in a group, such as self-disclosure, giving and receiving feedback,
etc.

therapists were trained in longer-term psychodynamic models, but
more recently there has been a growth of more focused, time-
limited models within the psychodynamic perspective and from a
variety of other theoretical perspectives as well.

■ WHY GROUPS?

There is now abundant evidence that psychotherapy groups are effective and that they are as effective or, in some cases, more effective than individual therapies (McRoberts et al. 1998; Tillitski
1990). Group therapies are also an efficient and cost-effective way
to deliver mental health services (Toseland and Siporin 1986). In
addition to these practical matters, however, group therapies offer
particular advantages. As mentioned before, therapy groups make
use of the powerful therapeutic tool of the group itself. There are
significant therapeutic factors that are inherent in the group setting.
Yalom (1994), in his classic text, delineated 11 therapeutic factors
operating in group psychotherapy. Scheidlinger (1997) combined
these with factors described by Bloch and Crouch (1985) and described 13 factors (see Table 8–1).

　　These factors are thought to be operating in all groups, independent of theory and technique. By themselves, these factors are

---

TABLE 8–1. **Therapeutic group factors**

Acceptance (sense of belonging, being accepted and valued by group and/ or individuals, "holding environment")

Universality ("being in same boat," "we are all in this together," "my problems are not unique")

Catharsis (ventilation of feelings, emotional release)

Corrective emotional experience (reliving earlier dysphoric emotional states with better outcomes)

Family transferences (parents, siblings, group-as-a-whole)

Modeling (emulation, identification with therapist and/or peers)

Reality testing (correcting misperceptions)

Learning from interpersonal interactions (feedback regarding one's behavior and its impact on others)

Vicarious learning (experiencing through empathic identification with others)

Insight ("meaning attribution"; interpersonal, intrapsychic, genetic)

Help from peers (altruism)

Guidance (imparting of information)

Instillation of hope (countering demoralization)

Note. This list follows factors described by Bloch and Crouch (1985) and Yalom (1994). Therapeutic group factors are differentiated from "conditions for change" and "therapeutic techniques" and defined as assumed "processes occurring in group therapy that contribute to the improvement of the patient's condition and are regarded as a function of the actions of the therapist, the other members of the group and the patient himself" (Bloch et al. 1981, p. 519). Some or all of these factors can operate together on conscious and/or unconscious levels; that is, "dynamic-contemporaneous" and "genetic-regressive" levels (Scheidlinger 1982).

Source. Reprinted from Scheidlinger S: "Group Dynamics and Group Psychotherapy Revisited: Four Decades Later." *International Journal of Group Psychotherapy* 47:155, 1997. Copyright 1997, Guilford Press. Used with permission.

believed to contribute to the improvement of patients in group therapy. Particularly noteworthy is Yalom's (1994) emphasis on the group as a social microcosm and a place for interpersonal learning. Interpersonal relationships are seen as fundamental in psychological development and therefore in psychological well-being. The group setting provides a unique opportunity, not just to talk about relationships, but to experience them in vivo. Although this possibility exists in individual therapy, the group setting provides a wider array of potential relationships and a more level playing field on which to interact. This allows for the diffusion of potential transference to the leader and the possibility of developing multiple transferences. Group members can also use the group setting as a relatively safe environment for learning new ways of relating and for experimenting with new behaviors. Another particular feature of group therapy is as an antidote to the debilitating affect of shame that appears to have so ubiquitous a role in psychopathology. Alonso and Rutan (1988) have discussed the particular advantages of group therapy for the resolution of shame, suggesting that the group climate provides a powerful opportunity for empathic mirroring and acceptance. There is little substitute for the healing power of the accepting, supportive, and cohesive community.

■ WHY TIME-LIMITED GROUPS?

We have already noted that group therapy is an efficient and cost-effective treatment modality. The substantial evidence that time-limited group therapy is effective, combined with the additional resource savings, suggests that these groups can be viewed as even more economical (Piper and Joyce 1996). In addition to cost savings, however, there are several potential therapeutic advantages of the use of time limits in group therapy. To begin with, potential patients can perceive time-limited groups as more manageable and therefore may be more likely to commit for the circumscribed period of time. As discussed in Chapter 3 for individual therapy, the time limit itself can produce an intensely evocative experience by highlighting the existential issues of time and meaning (Mann 1973). The consistent acknowledgment of the finiteness of time can instigate and inspire the group process. The time limits can also decrease the development of prolonged dependency on the therapy and can reduce the likelihood of harmful regression (Budman et al. 1996a). The imposition of a time limit may also be useful in helping patients move beyond a victim stance by promoting a greater sense of personal agency.

Time-limited group therapy is different from more open-ended therapy in a number of significant ways (see Chapter 1). MacKenzie (1990) has enumerated some of these distinctions, which are in basic agreement with those drawn earlier by Klein (1985) and Poey (1985). What is essential in all accounts of time-limited group therapies is the emphasis on the time limit, therapist activity, focus and goal setting, and the selection and preparation of group members.

■ GROUP DYNAMICS AND GROUP THERAPY

Group therapies vary with respect to the degree of attention paid to the process, as opposed to the content, of the group. They also vary according to whether the interventions of the therapist are focused predominantly on the individual members, on dyads or subgroups, or on the group as a whole. To maximize the potential of any group therapy, however, a working knowledge of group dynamics is essential. To make the most of the treatment modality, the group therapist must possess an understanding of how all groups function, regardless of the type of group or the theoretical perspective. A number of specific factors are common to the dynamics of all small groups. These include group boundaries, group norms, group roles, group cohesion, and stages of group development. Scheidlinger (1997) asserts his belief in the inseparability of individual and group dynamics. One of the interesting and considerably challenging aspects of group work is the constant shifting of attention between the dynamics of the individual group members to those of the group as a whole. A more complete discussion of group dynamics is beyond the scope of this chapter, but the interested reader can find thorough treatment of the subject throughout the literature (e.g., Scheidlinger 1997).

■ TYPES OF GROUPS AND THEORETICAL PERSPECTIVES

Group therapy encompasses a wide array of groups and treatment modalities derived from a range of theoretical perspectives.

Scheidlinger (2000) has described 12 distinct major models of group psychotherapy that were in existence by 1980, at least half of which can be considered broadly psychodynamic. MacKenzie (1990) discussed six different theoretical perspectives for establishing an interpersonal focus for group treatment. Current group therapies range theoretically from psychodynamic and interpersonally oriented perspectives to cognitive and behavioral perspectives. Groups are used for a wide array of problems with a wide range of patients across the diagnostic spectrum. Groups can be vehicles for psychoeducation and skills training or can be directed toward uncovering and understanding interpersonal or intrapsychic dynamics. There are groups based on specific diagnostic criteria (e.g., bulimia, panic disorder, depression, medical illness), groups formed around specific situational or developmental issues (e.g., bereavement, divorce, middle age), and more general interpersonal groups.

Broadly speaking, group therapy modalities vary along a number of conceptually inexact but potentially useful continua. These continua can be construed as deriving from theoretical distinctions to some degree, but they are perhaps better thought of as deriving from consideration of the basic purposes and goals of the particular groups. To begin with, the group therapies vary along what has been termed a supportive-interpretive or supportive-expressive continuum (MacKenzie 1997). This is similar to the early distinction made by Sifneos (1971/1996) regarding anxiety-suppressive versus anxiety-provoking short-term individual therapies. One end of the spectrum emphasizes the provision of direct and practical support, whereas the other end brings the expectation of intensive exploration and emotional expression. On the interpretive end of the continuum, the treatment focuses on affective expression and gaining insight into underlying interpersonal or intrapsychic dynamics. Although the therapist's stance is less directive and more neutral regarding the internal conflicts, defenses are actively confronted, challenged, and interpreted, and increased anxiety is expected as an inevitable consequence of the more probing therapeutic technique. Transference is actively explored and interpreted.

Groups also vary with respect to the degree to which they focus on interpersonal interactions. For example, in Yalom's (1994) interpersonal therapy groups, the focus on here-and-now interactions is viewed as the primary therapeutic agent, whereas these interactions do not become a primary focus in cognitive or behaviorally oriented groups. All groups make use of the interpersonal context of the group setting, but on the behavioral end of the continuum it is a vehicle for encouragement, reinforcement, modeling, and so forth, whereas on the interpersonal end, treatment focuses specifically on the nature of the interactions.

Other dimensions in which group therapies vary are the extent to which the therapist's interventions are directed to individual group members or to the group as a whole and whether they are directed to changing specific behaviors, interpersonal patterns, or intrapsychic dynamics. Debates continue in the literature over the centrality of any of these dimensions (Scheidlinger 1997). The dimensions discussed here represent only a few along which group therapies vary, and like many sets of distinctions, they eventually break down in the reality of therapeutic practice. This breakdown, along with empirical research indicating that treatments from different theoretical perspectives tend to get similar results, may account in some measure for the clear trend in the field toward a greater degree of integration.

This trend toward integration is seen in the time-effective group therapy model proposed by Budman and Gurman (1988). The model is fundamentally interpersonal in nature, but it incorporates aspects of existential theory and is set in an adult developmental context. Budman borrows from Yalom (1994) and Mann (1973) and provides a developmental context in which interpersonal and existential factors are understood. The approach also incorporates supportive elements and aspects of what have been termed *competency-based models* (Friedman 1997). Time-limited treatments of any type, and time-limited groups in particular, are viewed from the perspective of an episodic treatment model. These groups are seen as part of a larger constellation of therapeutic experiences over the course of a patient's life span. The work emphasizes limited and achievable goals and catalyzing a process of change that will extend beyond the therapy. The model has received empirical support and is a widely regarded clinical model of brief therapy. What follows is largely adapted from the exposition of this model in *Theory and Practice of Brief Therapy* (Budman and Gurman 1988).

■ AN ILLUSTRATIVE MODEL OF TIME-LIMITED GROUP PSYCHOTHERAPY

Interpersonal-Developmental-Existential Approach to Time-Limited Group Psychotherapy

In the interpersonal-developmental-existential model, psychological disturbance is understood as occurring within a context of interpersonal dysfunction and developmental desynchrony. Group therapy attempts to optimize the therapeutic factors that are uniquely available in the group setting by actively facilitating the development of group process, group cohesion, interpersonal interaction and relationship, self-disclosure, and the exchange of feedback. Several of the fundamental underpinnings of the model are summarized in Table 8–2.

The establishment of the duration of the group, like many of the other technical aspects of the model, is viewed as a function of the specific focus and purpose of the particular group. The general rule of thumb is that the duration ought to be the shortest period of time necessary to achieve the goals of the group. The time limit of a relatively circumscribed, crisis-oriented group thus may be 8 sessions, whereas that of a group focused on developmental life transition issues, such as young adulthood or midlife, may be 15 sessions, and a group focused on chronic and pervasive interpersonal difficulties may have a limit of 60–70 sessions. The thrust, then, is toward time-consciousness and time-effectiveness rather than mere brevity.

Because space does not permit a full discussion of all the foregoing factors, we confine our discussion here to elaborating on the establishment and maintenance of an interpersonal focus, the

TABLE 8–2. **Characteristics of the interpersonal-developmental-existential model of time-limited group therapy**

1. Establishing and maintaining an interpersonal focus in the group
2. Active therapist stance
3. Emphasis on group interaction and group cohesiveness
4. Existential factors and the use of time limits
5. Pregroup screening and preparation

Source. Adapted from Budman and Gurman 1988 and Budman et al. 1996a.

screening and preparation of potential group members, stages of group development, and some technical considerations in running groups.

Focus

Establishing a clearly defined focus is absolutely essential for any successful time-limited therapy but can be particularly challenging to achieve in a group. It is the job of the group therapist to be clear about the focus and goals of the group and to be able to articulate these explicitly to potential group members and potential referral sources. The group therapist straddles the line between foci that are too narrowly defined and so pertain too specifically to any particular individual, and those that are too general and thereby apply so loosely to everyone that they lack vitality or meaning.

Budman and Gurman (1988) recommend a working focus that is interpersonal and imbedded in a context of adult development rather than choosing a symptom or diagnostic focus. They maintain that interpersonal foci allow for optimal use of the unique aspects of the group experience and foster the group as a social microcosm in which to examine old patterns of behavior and experiment with new ones. For example, if one considers the developmental stage of young adulthood, the relevant interpersonal concerns often pertain to the capacity and willingness to form intimate relationships. This becomes the focus for the group, and a number of important decisions, such as group composition, size, and duration, then flow from this choice. Potential group members must be helped to understand or construe their presenting issues through the lens of the interpersonal focus. (This topic is discussed further under "Screening and Pregroup Preparation" later in this chapter.)

Through establishment of the focus of the group, the homogeneity of the group membership begins to develop. Unlike many models of longer-term group therapy that encourage some degree of heterogeneity to achieve a broader range of interpersonal exchange, this model of time-limited therapy strives to achieve greater homogeneity. Homogeneity allows for more rapid coalescing of the group and therefore for more rapid development of universality and cohesion. Understandably, this rapid development of cohesion is necessary in a group that does not have time to allow such cohesion to evolve at its own pace.

Homogeneity can be achieved along a number of dimensions, from the concrete (e.g., the age of the members) to the more abstract (e.g., core conflicts of individuals). Two particularly important dimensions are the homogeneity of the group members' coping capacities (ego strength) and the homogeneity of the group's purpose. Group members must be relatively similar in their capacities to navigate through life's stresses and to tolerate the potential discomfort generated in the group, and they must have a similar sense of purpose for being in the group. Homogeneity of purpose is achieved through the definition and acceptance of the group's focus. For example, a depressed young adult who is focused on somatic complaints and is unable or unwilling to explore the interpersonal contributions to and consequences of his or her depression is unlikely to do well in this group.

Screening and Pregroup Preparation

Although careful screening and preparation are important for any group therapy, they are essential for time-limited groups. Given the constraint of time, it is vital to have formed a group that can hit the ground running. A time-limited group cannot afford the dropouts or the considerable lag time to get going that a longer-term group might be able to withstand. In certain respects, the process of screening and preparation are intertwined. The process of assessing whether a patient will be an appropriate group member involves a collaborative effort of reframing the presenting concerns and negotiating an interpersonal focus, which is also part of preparing a patient for group. In addition, formulating an individual focus that is consistent with the group's principal focus and gaining the patient's agreement to pursue these foci is both a selection and a preparation process. Screening and preparation require open, collaborative dialogue that is focused on interpersonal meaning in terms of both personal history and the group process.

Even in the present sophisticated consumer market, most people know very little about group therapy except for the often inaccurate information they are able to glean from the popular media. People tend to be leery of group therapy, sometimes confusing it with self-help groups, encounter groups, or est. Often patients, and even many therapists, tend to view group therapy as watered down or second rate. In many ways, pregroup preparation can be said to begin at the referral source. If the referring agent perceives group therapy as a powerful tool, then that message is conveyed to the patient. On the other hand, if group treatment is viewed as a cheap but second-rate alternative, then the opportunity for the patient to a have positive therapeutic experience is greatly diminished.

One question that arises is whether screening and preparation should be conducted individually or in a group. Budman and Gurman (1988) recommend a combination of both. They suggest at least some brief individual contact with the group leader and a group screening and preparation workshop (see "Pregroup Workshop" later in this section).

Selection

Budman and Gurman (1988) suggest that selection criteria for their time-limited groups follow from the purpose and focus of the particular group and will therefore vary. Although they maintain that most patients can benefit from some form of time-limited group treatment, a discussion of general inclusion and exclusion guidelines may be helpful to the reader.

General exclusion criteria tend to be active psychosis; paranoid, schizoid, or sociopathic character pathology; active substance abuse; active suicidal or homicidal ideation; strict externalizing and somaticizing; and excessively disorganized, withdrawn, rageful, or monopolizing behavior. Inclusion criteria include a minimum ability to relate, a significant degree of motivation to join the group, and the ability to articulate a focal area of difficulty that is essentially interpersonal in nature. Klein (1985) summarizes selection by stating that the most important factor is congruence between the identified goals and tasks of the group and the ego capacity and motivation of the member to accomplish them.

Individual Screening Interview

The individual screening interview generally lasts between 30 minutes and 1 hour and is used to accomplish a number of important functions. The interview assists in the assessment process, provides information to the patient about groups in general and about the particular group, initiates a bond between the therapist and the potential group member, and provides an opportunity to frame the patient's concerns in a form that is conducive to making optimal use of the group experience. The therapist needs to help the patient to articulate an individual focus, to tie that focus to the focus of the group, and to articulate circumscribed, achievable goals. It is also very useful during this interview to help prospective group members to predict repetitive patterns that are likely to emerge in the group and relevant obstacles to achieving their goals. These predictions can serve as red flags to which both the patient and the therapist can attend.

Clinical Example

Tom, a dysthymic 27-year-old, single man, was referred to a young adult group within a large health maintenance organization (HMO). When asked during the pregroup interview about his reason for seeking treatment, Tom responded that he had been "kind of down" and that his girlfriend said it had been affecting their relationship. He said the person who saw him for an intake interview suggested that this group might be helpful and that he was willing to "give it a shot." The leader had advertised the group as a group for men and women between the ages of 21 and 35 who are struggling with intimacy and emotional closeness in relationships.

The group leader pursued the following line of inquiry, attempting to establish a possible interpersonal individual focus:

Leader: You say you've been feeling down, but your girlfriend sent you.

Tom: Yes, she said that I seemed so emotionally cut off and distant and that it's affecting the relationship.

Leader: Is that true?

Tom: I don't know. Probably.

Leader: Probably?

Tom: Yeah, I guess. Half the time I don't really know what I'm feeling.

Leader: Well, I would imagine that's part of what your girlfriend might be getting at.

Tom: I suppose so, but you know, when I was a kid, we were taught to just suck it up and get on with things. I'm not sure I want to tell her everything on my mind.

Leader: Is it possible that just "sucking it up" is contributing to feeling down and to this distance between you and your girlfriend as well?

Here the leader is tying the patient's presenting concern about his mood to an interpersonal style and framing it in such a way as to be understood interpersonally. After establishing this connection and making sure the patient is able to absorb it, the leader can go on to link the individual focus with the focus of the group and assess the patient's interest in pursuing that focus.

Leader: That is something many people your age struggle with. Sometimes it's hard to know what you're feeling, and

> sometimes even if you know, it's hard to share it. But that
> seems to create all sorts of problems for you, particularly
> by isolating you from your girlfriend. Is that something
> you can imagine yourself beginning to work on in this
> group?

A statement like this one begins to establish a sense of universality, links the individual concern with the larger group focus, and attempts to assess the patient's interest in pursuing this group theme. This process of honing the individual focus and framing it to match the focus of the group is an essential aspect of the screening and preparation process. By the end of the interview, the patient ought to have a greater sense of the purpose of the group and how his or her individual purpose does or does not fit with it.

Pregroup Workshop

The individual contact with the potential group member is necessary but probably insufficient for either selection or preparation of group members. The best predictor of actual in-group behavior is a sample of that behavior. To that end, Budman and Gurman (1988) recommend a pregroup workshop, which takes place a week or two before the start date of the group. This workshop is used to better assess potential members for the group and to familiarize and prepare them for the group experience.

The therapist begins the workshop by explaining both the similarities and the differences between the workshop and the actual group. The therapist explains that the purpose of the workshop is to familiarize the members with group processes and to determine goodness of fit with the group, but he or she also makes it clear that the actual group therapy will be far less structured than the workshop. This switch to a less structured format can be difficult and has caused some to question the use of a workshop (Piper et al. 1992), but Budman and Gurman (1988) believe that the benefits clearly outweigh any potential drawbacks. For example, the use of such workshops has been shown to reduce subsequent dropout rates (Budman et al. 1981; Piper et al. 1979).

The components of the workshop include 1) introductions in dyads, 2) a subgroup task that varies depending on the central focus of the group, and 3) a whole-group exercise. The therapist looks for problematic behavior, such as excessive withdrawal or aggressive, paranoid, or monopolistic behavior. The therapist encourages, facilitates, and reinforces desirable group behaviors, such as appropriate self-disclosure and the exchange of feedback. At the end of the workshop, the therapist summarizes the experience and asks the patients to consider whether they want to commit to the group. The members then contact the therapist with their decisions unless the therapist needs to advise a patient against joining the group.

Technical Considerations

The group leader assumes a very active therapeutic stance from the outset of the group, which includes jump-starting the group when necessary, drawing in group members, setting limits on behaviors that may be harmful to the group, and tying themes back to the central focus of the group (Budman et al. 1996a). However, this stance is not intended to be confused with a coercive or confrontational position. Emphasis is placed on the facilitation of the group interaction and the power of the group members to help one another. Interventions may be directed toward an individual, a subgroup, or the group as a whole, depending on the need and the stage of the group. Budman urges therapists to remain flexible in their technical interventions and not to rely on procrustean, one-size-fits-all concepts. The focus is on the interpersonal rather than the intrapsychic and on conscious and preconscious material. In general, defenses are not actively challenged or interpreted; rather, the interpersonal patterns and their consequences are explored and alternatives are discussed. The emphasis of the model is on behavioral and emotional change through experiential learning rather than on insight through interpretation.

This active, directive, and supportive stance is certainly a departure from the neutrality and abstinence of the traditional psychoanalytic approach. Budman and his colleagues (1996a) question the utility and even the possibility of therapeutic neutrality and maintain the necessity of these modifications to adapt to the time limitation. However, they recognize the potential constraints that this approach may place on certain processes, especially transference to the group leader. They accept that a rapid positive transference to the leader and the group is desirable. However, unlike Piper et al. (1992), who practice from a position that is considerably more traditionally psychodynamic, Budman and his colleagues deemphasize the role of transference, and transference interpretations in particular. The focus is on the conscious here-and-now and there-and-now relationships. The past is deemphasized, and historical material is invoked only insofar as it clearly illuminates the present and future (Budman et al. 1994).

Group cohesion is viewed as an essential component of successful group therapy. It can be thought of as conceptually similar to the therapeutic alliance in individual therapy. For the therapy group to do its work, it must come together and create a safe and productive unit. For time-limited groups, this coalescing must occur relatively rapidly. Budman conceives of cohesiveness as a multidimensional and dynamic construct that includes elements of trust, involvement, cooperation, and caring and that may mean different things depending on the stage of the group. What contributes to cohesion at the beginning of the group may not do so during the middle or end phases. For example, discussing material from outside the group is associated with high levels of cohesion early in the group, whereas discussing material from inside the group is associated with higher cohesion at later stages of the group (Budman et al. 1994).

Stages of Group Development

All theories of group processes describe stages of group development. As groups progress from the beginning, through the middle, and to termination, different work takes place requiring different types of therapist involvement. Budman and Gurman (1988) propose five stages of group development: 1) starting the group, 2) early therapy, 3) middle of the group, 4) late therapy, and 5) termination.

They also recommend a 6-month follow-up session, which they suggest may constitute a sixth stage. These stages roughly correspond to those proposed by MacKenzie (1997): engagement, differentiation, interpersonal work, and termination.

Here we focus on the beginning of the group, the middle phase (including the *group crisis*), the late or "working" group, and the termination. We discuss the characteristic group phenomena and particular technical considerations that pertain to these stages. We also provide clinical material from a young adult interpersonal group to illustrate the work that is done during a given stage.

Beginning and Early Group (Engagement)

In a standard group of 12–15 sessions, the beginning phase may constitute 2–4 sessions. The basic concerns of the group during this stage are safety and acceptance, boundaries and rules, and the roles that will be assumed by the leader and the group members. These major concerns provide the backdrop of the group until someone emerges as the "patient." The leader begins by stating the rules and contract of the group, including the boundaries of membership, time, confidentiality, and appropriate behavior. The leader also reiterates the focus and goals of the group.

The major task of the group during this phase is cohesion. The leader's role is to facilitate this cohesion by encouraging the development of universality and fostering acceptance. The leader invites participation directly and facilitates the group interaction. The technical emphasis is on pointing out similarities among the group members, making joining statements, focusing on emergent themes, and tying those themes to the group focus. The leader wants to contain premature or inappropriate self-disclosures. An important aspect of technique involves the leader's summary statements, which are generally made toward the end of the sessions. These statements are used to bind each session together, to connect the sessions with one another, and to tie the sessions to the group focus.

It is important during this stage to be aware of possible screening errors that may have been made and that must be addressed in a timely fashion. For example, extremely monopolistic or decompensating individuals must be managed or removed from the group. The issue of time appears to be a remote concern during this stage, but the leader must maintain the awareness of the time limit by consistently reminding the group at each session of the number of sessions remaining. As the group moves through this engagement period and early group development, the members begin to address the issues for which they came, at first superficially and gradually more deeply.

Clinical Examples

Engaging Members and Building Cohesiveness
Tom: I'm having a hard time really saying what I feel about that.
Leader: Joan, you also mentioned some similar difficulties in here. Are there other people feeling that way?

Defining Roles and Responsibilities
Steve: *(to the leader)* So what are your goals for us?
Leader: I certainly can share my vision for the group, but even more importantly, I wonder what goals the group sees for itself.

Summary Statements
Leader: It makes sense that today the group is grappling with questions about how safe it is in here, what's appropriate to talk about, and how much to invest in these relationships that will only last for 12 weeks. Certainly this is understandable, given where we are in the group. But I also wonder if this doesn't speak to some of the larger concerns about intimacy and commitment to relationships that brought you all here to this group in the first place.

Middle Group (Differentiation)

As the group moves past the early engagement and heads into the middle stage of development, a growing sense of frustration and even discord can arise. This has been referred to as the group crisis.

Group theorists and researchers agree that this is an important phase of the group whose successful negotiation can lead to a deepening of the group's work. MacKenzie (1990, 1997) characterizes this as a stage of differentiation where, once the group has coalesced into a secure unit, it must allow for the separateness and individuality of its members. Budman and Gurman (1988) focus more on the growing discontent of the members about not accomplishing what they set out to accomplish and the increasing recognition of the limited time. The dissatisfaction can be overt or sometimes subtle and covert and can be directly focused on the leader or displaced onto others. Sometimes the crisis is connected to the focus of the group— such as a flight from deepening relationships or an inability to commit if one can't have it all in a young adult group—but sometimes the focus must be temporarily set aside to address the immediate crisis. What is essential is that the leader confront the crisis directly, openly, and nondefensively. The crisis can evoke powerful countertransferential feelings, such as shame, inadequacy, disappointment, or even rage in the leader. Budman and Gurman (1988) emphasize that the leader must remain calm and be able to recognize, acknowledge, and address the crisis when it emerges. If it is ignored or avoided, depression and helplessness can set in, but if the crisis is successfully addressed, the group moves to higher levels of cohesion and greater depth. MacKenzie (1997) suggests that the group needs to be able to be positively and constructively confrontational and that members learn this by being more challenging of each other but also by collectively confronting the leader.

Clinical Example

Joan: *(referring to an outside relationship)* I still keep going back, even though I know it's not going to be good for me.

Steve: We've been talking about this for a few weeks now and you don't seem to be getting anywhere. Is this helping you? Because, I'm not sure. I mean we go over and over this.

Tom: We can't say what's helpful.

Steve: Well, she's not taking our advice.

Leader: It's sounding terribly frustrating.

Steve: Well, I think we need more direction to get somewhere.

Leader: I wonder if other people may not be feeling that too.

Joan: I sort of feel that at times. I want to know what you think. I'm not sure I'd do it, but I want to know your opinions.

Leader: I can understand that sometimes it must be pretty frustrating in here thinking that I have the answers but I'm not giving them, or that we're running out of time and there's still a lot we haven't accomplished. But the truth is that I don't have all the answers and we won't accomplish everything in here. But maybe we can still accomplish something, and maybe you have considerably more to give to each other than you think.

In this example, the leader does not ignore or avoid the negative affect but addresses it directly, while reflecting on the reality of the situation with which the members must struggle.

Late Group (Interpersonal Work)

If the prior stages have been successfully negotiated, the group now really hits its stride. Time is running out, and extra effort is required to get the work accomplished before it's too late. The group members are more ready and able to take risks, and concerns and emotions are expressed at more profound and connected levels. Group tasks involve exploring interpersonal patterns more deeply and experimenting with new behaviors in the group. The leader must maintain the focus against drift or overexpansion. The issue of loss will begin to emerge, which will be addressed more fully in the next stage.

Clinical Example

Tom: I got laid off last week and I haven't been able to tell anyone. I saw my family over the weekend, but I couldn't tell them.

Leader: I wonder what made it possible to tell this family?

Tom: I feel like that's why we're here, and, I don't know, I trust them. We all have problems and they'll listen.

Steve [*breaks in*]: You know what you have to do is get the resume right out. There's still a lot going on out there. When I'm down, the best thing to do is get right back out there.

Leader: Tom, how are you feeling right now about Steve's comments?

Tom: I know what kinds of things I need to do. That's not really what I'm looking for. I just need someone to listen or to say, "that sucks." That's what I never got growing up. I just want to hear, "Are you OK?" [*starts to tear up*]

Steve [*spontaneously*]: I'm sorry, you're right. I know I do that.

Leader: That must have been hard for you to say, Tom, and [*to Steve*] hard for you to hear. Maybe it's OK not to have all the solutions, but just to listen and care…but that can be hard.

In this example, the leader highlights a pattern in Steve's relationships of binding his anxiety with problem solving. Tom is helped to ask for what he needs and to begin to feel his emotions. Ultimately, Tom gets what he's asking for from the group, Steve examines an important interpersonal pattern, and the group moves to a deeper, more connected place.

Termination

The termination stage is an enormously important phase of the group. It can be intensely emotional and powerful for everyone. Termination forces the group to struggle with the existential issues of finiteness, not only of time but of accomplishment, of individual responsibility (going it alone), and of the inescapable reality of loss.

The reactions to termination can vary. Some members may react as though it's a surprise: "Is next week the last session?" Others may attempt to prolong the group: "If we only had another four sessions," or "Let's plan weekly meetings on our own." Still others may begin to disparage the group as a way to assuage the pain of loss. Again, the leader's countertransference may be evoked, stirring up past losses and disappointments, feelings of inadequacy, or rescue fantasies. The leader must remain aware of his or her own feelings and must stay positively focused. The task of termination is to review and consolidate the group's accomplishments, to face the loss together, and to find a way to say goodbye. Often the termination can be nicely woven into the focus of the group. For example, in the young adult group, finding new ways of coping with loss allows for greater intimacy. The members experience the possibility of separation while still feeling closeness and connection.

Clinical Example

Aretha: Unfortunately, I won't be able to be here for the last group.

Tom: What's going on?

Aretha: I had this business trip planned for a while, and I tried to get out of it but I can't.

Jack: Sometimes those things happen.

Joan: You did what you can, so don't feel bad.

Leader: It's very hard to say goodbye.

Aretha: I knew you were going to say that. I knew you would make a big deal out of it, but I tried. You know it isn't really fair that we have to stop just because the HMO says so.

Leader: So, maybe there is a wish in the group that we wouldn't have to say goodbye.

Tom: We can all get together sometimes after the end, if we want.

Leader: Well, of course that's true, but this group will no longer "be" after our last meeting. And the fact is, we need to find a way to face that together, hopefully in a way that's different and better than many of the goodbyes you've all experienced before.

In this example, the group leader focuses the group on the task of facing the emotions associated with loss and finding a better way to say goodbye. To ensure a therapeutic resolution, the leader cannot be seduced by the pull of the group or by his or her own countertransferential needs to avoid the loss.

■ EMPIRICAL FINDINGS

The effectiveness of this model has been tested in several clinical trials. Budman et al. (1984) found that patients in short-term group therapy showed significantly greater improvement than did control subjects on a waiting list, especially with regard to target symptomatology. These differences, however, were not evident at 6-month follow-up, a finding that the authors attribute to the additional therapy both groups received in that interim period.

Budman et al. (1988) compared time-limited group therapy with time-limited individual therapy. Patients in both conditions improved significantly. Although there were no significant differences between the types of treatment, patients reported a preference for individual therapy. Budman et al. (1996b) performed an uncontrolled study of the effectiveness of this model, using time-limited but not short-term groups of 72 sessions with patients with character disorders. They found that patients who completed the groups reported significant improvement in symptomatology and self-esteem; however, the study suffered from a high dropout rate and the lack of a control group.

More generally, a number of reviews of the group therapy literature and meta-analyses of the data have indicated clear and robust support for the efficacy of group therapy. Toseland and Siporin's (1986) review of the literature led them to conclude that group therapy is at least as effective as individual therapy, and in 25% of the studies they reviewed it was more effective. Tillitski (1990) performed a meta-analysis of studies in which group therapy and individual therapy were compared with a control condition and found equivalent effects for both modalities. Piper and Joyce (1996) conducted a rigorous review of group therapy studies that met stringent methodological criteria. Although the large majority of group therapies studied in the literature can be considered time limited, Piper and Joyce (1996) confined their analysis only to groups of 6 months or less in duration. Overall, the results of their review were consistent with those of previous reviews, indicating support for the efficacy of group therapy and the relative equivalence of group and individual treatments from a variety of theoretical perspectives and for a wide range of patients. They do, however, point out that in a number of studies no significant differences were found between patients receiving group therapy and control subjects on particular outcome measures, and so time-limited group therapy should not be seen as a panacea for all types of problems (Piper and Joyce 1996). They suggest that determining the limitations as well as the successes is the necessary path of future research.

■ RELEVANCE FOR MANAGED CARE

Given the efficacy and efficiency of time-limited group therapy, its role in a managed care system can be enormous. Most time-limited groups fit well within the standard 20-session limits of many managed care systems, and they can reduce the percentage of staff time devoted to nonemergency patient care. MacKenzie (1994, 1997, 2000) maintains that time-limited groups ought to play a significant role as part of a comprehensive group therapy program within any future mental health service delivery system. He suggests that such a comprehensive group program needs to provide a range of groups designed to address different levels of clinical need. Such a program should include time-limited groups designed for crisis intervention, lasting up to approximately eight sessions and comprising 12–26 session groups. These groups should be designed to focus on specific diagnostic criteria, such as panic disorder or bulimia; situational disturbances, such as bereavement or divorce; psychoeducation and skills building, such as management of stress or medical disease; and, finally, general interpersonal groups. The program also ought to include longer-term groups for patients who require ongoing care.

Although the potential advantages of such a program appear obvious, there have been a number of obstacles to the implementation of these group programs within managed care systems, resulting in their underuse (MacKenzie 2000; Rosenberg and Zimet 1995; Steenbarger and Budman 1996). Among the barriers discussed in the literature are attitudinal factors, such as patient and therapist biases against group treatment, and structural/institutional factors, such as patient benefit structures, clinician compensation protocols, and the difficult logistics of establishing time-limited groups. Errors are made by systems that either attempt to overuse group therapy by assigning everyone to groups regardless of need or that institutionally discourage any use of group treatment. An additional factor limiting the expansion of the use of group therapy is the training of therapists. Many therapists have not been adequately trained in group therapy, and of those who have received training, even fewer are well trained in time-effective modalities. These limitations have led some to conclude that the routine use of group therapy as a primary therapeutic modality may still be in the distance (Piper and Joyce 1996).

Scheidlinger (2000), reflecting on the state of group therapy at the millennium, predicted that most treatment groups in the public sector are likely to be time limited and, given their proven effectiveness and cost-efficiency, these groups are likely to prosper. Several others have suggested that certain conditions need to be met to foster that prosperity (MacKenzie 2000; Steenbarger and Budman 1996). These conditions include a better-informed consumer, better-trained clinicians, and a health care system that has been educated about the clear benefits of group therapy.

■ REFERENCES

Alonso A, Rutan S: The experience of shame and the restoration of self-respect in group therapy. Int J Group Psychother 38:3–27, 1988

Bloch S, Crouch E: Therapeutic Factors in Group Psychotherapy. Oxford, England, Oxford University Press, 1985

Bloch S., Crouch E, Reibstein J: Therapeutic factors in group psychotherapy: a review. Arch Gen Psychiatry 38:519–526, 1981

Budman SH, Gurman AS: Theory and Practice of Brief Therapy. New York, Guilford, 1988

Budman SH, Clifford M, Bader L, et al: Experiential pre-group preparation and screening. Group 5:19–26, 1981

Budman SH, Demby A, Feldstein M, et al: The effects of time-limited group psychotherapy: a controlled study. Int J Group Psychother 34:587–603, 1984

Budman SH, Demby A, Redondo JP, et al: Comparative outcome in time-limited individual and group psychotherapy. Int J Group Psychother 38:63–86, 1988

Budman SH, Simeone PG, Reilly R, et al: Progress in short-term and time-limited group psychotherapy: evidence and implications, in Handbook of Group Psychotherapy: an Empirical and Clinical Synthesis. Edited by Fuhriman A, Burlingame GM. New York, Wiley, 1994, pp 319–339

Budman SH, Cooley S, Demby A, et al: A model of time-effective group psychotherapy for patients with personality disorders: the clinical model. Int J Group Psychother 46:329–355, 1996a

Budman SH, Demby A, Soldz S, et al: Time-limited group psychotherapy for patients with personality disorders: outcomes and dropouts. Int J Group Psychother 46:357–377, 1996b

Friedman S: Time-effective Psychotherapy. Boston, MA, Allyn and Bacon, 1997

Klein R: Some principles of short-term group therapy. Int J Group Psychother 35:309–329, 1985

MacKenzie KR: Introduction to Time-Limited Group Psychotherapy. Washington, DC, American Psychiatric Association, 1990

MacKenzie KR: Where is here and when is now? the adaptational challenge of mental health reform for group psychotherapy. Int J Group Psychother 44:407–428, 1994

MacKenzie KR: Time-Managed Group Psychotherapy: Effective Clinical Applications. Washington, DC, American Psychiatric Association, 1997

MacKenzie KR: Group psychotherapies and managed care, in A Psychologist's Proactive Guide to Managed Mental Health Care. Edited by Kent AJ, Hersen M. Mahwah, NJ, Lawrence Erlbaum Associates, 2000

Mann J: Time-Limited Psychotherapy. Cambridge, MA, Harvard University Press, 1973

Marsh CL: Group treatment of the psychoses by the psychological equivalent of revival. Mental Hygiene 15:328–349, 1909

McRoberts C, Burlingame GM, Hoag MJ: Comparative efficacy of individual and group psychotherapy: a meta-analytic perspective. Group Dyn 2:101–117, 1998

Piper WE, Joyce AS: A consideration of factors influencing the utilization of time-limited short-term group psychotherapy. Int J Group Psychother 46:311–328, 1996

Piper WE, Debbane EG, Garant J, et al: Pretraining for group psychotherapy: a cognitive-experiential approach. Arch Gen Psychiatry 36:1250–1256, 1979

Piper WE, McCallum M, Azim HFA: Adaptation to Loss Through Short-Term Group Psychotherapy. New York, Guilford, 1992

Poey K: Guidelines for the practice of brief, dynamic group therapy. Int J Group Psychother 35:331–354, 1985

Pratt JH: The home sanatorium treatment of consumption. Boston Medical Surgery Journal 154:210–216, 1905

Rosenberg SA, Zimet CN: Brief group treatment and managed mental health care. Int J Group Psychother 45:367–379, 1995

Scheidlinger S: Focus on Group Psychotherapy: Clinical Essays. Madison, CT, International Universities Press, 1982

Scheidlinger S: Group dynamics and group psychotherapy revisited: four decades later. Int J Group Psychother 47:141–159, 1997

Scheidlinger S: The group psychotherapy movement at the millennium: some historical perspectives. Int J Group Psychother 50:315–339, 2000

Sifneos P: Two different kinds of psychotherapy of short duration (1971), in Essential Papers on Short-Term Dynamic Therapy. Edited by Groves J. New York, New York University Press, 1996

Steenbarger BN, Budman SH: Group psychotherapy and managed behavioral health care: current trends and future challenges. Int J Group Psychother 46:297–309, 1996

Tillitski CJ: A meta-analysis of estimated effect sizes for group versus individual control treatments. Int J Group Psychother 40:215–224, 1990

Toseland RW, Siporin M: When to recommend group treatment: a review of the clinical and the research literature. Int J Group Psychother 36:171–201, 1986

Yalom I: The Theory and Practice of Group Psychotherapy, 4th Edition. New York, Basic Books, 1994

9

THE RECIPROCAL RELATIONSHIP BETWEEN PHARMACOTHERAPY AND PSYCHOTHERAPY

> The future may teach us how to exercise a direct influence, by particular chemical substances, upon the amounts of energy and their distribution in the apparatus of the mind. It may be that there are undreamed possibilities of therapy....
>
> *Freud (1940/1964), p. 182*

Despite Freud's belief in the potential of psychoactive chemicals to aid psychoanalytic work, psychodynamic therapists have been relatively slow in using medications in their work. The appearance of this chapter in this book underscores the need for those providing brief dynamic therapy to consider the effective use of medications. In fact, the use of medications during psychotherapy fits quite comfortably within psychoanalytic tradition.

Before embarking on his psychological theories, Freud, about a century ago, was struggling to conceptualize the interrelationship between mind and brain in *Project for a Scientific Psychology* (Freud 1895/1966). As a neurologist, he recognized that brain pathology must have something to do with psychiatric disturbances. However, the limited knowledge of brain function available to him in the latter years of the nineteenth century sharply limited his theoretical speculations. Now, we are witnessing an explosion of knowledge about the brain. The time is ripe for a renewal of theoretical speculation about the neurology of psychotherapy.

Pharmacotherapy also fits comfortably with the search for meaning within the analytic tradition. Although many analysts have claimed that medication interfered with the development of the transference, they failed to note the possibility that medications themselves sometimes serve as oval or round blank screens for the projection of myriad idiosyncratic meanings. Purple or red, yellow or green, the little objects serve as variations of Rorschach inkblots that can illuminate patterns of cognitive, emotional, behavioral, and interpersonal dysfunction.

One could hope, then, that a tighter conceptual relationship between mind and brain, between pharmacotherapy and psychotherapy, could lead to more efficient and effective treatments. Research evidence is beginning to accumulate to suggest that combined treatments may be more effective than single treatments alone in the aggregate (Sperry 1995). However, no controlled studies have investigated the potential utility of incorporating the meaning of medications into the psychotherapeutic process or whether and how medications accelerate the psychotherapeutic process. These questions require innovative protocols yet to be developed. Instead, clinicians must rely on astute clinical observation to substantiate and develop the possibility that medications can accelerate the process of psychotherapeutic change, through both their direct pharmacological effects and their idiosyncratic meanings to individual patients.

The first section of this chapter addresses the beginnings of our understanding of the neurology of psychotherapy. It summarizes seminal research in obsessive-compulsive disorder that lays a foundation for solid clinical speculation about the convergent effects of pharmacotherapy and psychotherapy on the "worry circuit." The second section addresses the role medications can play across the stages of psychotherapy. In the third and fourth sections, several examples are offered to illustrate the manner in which reactions to pharmacotherapy reveal key patterns that are useful for psychotherapeutic understanding—a psychodynamics of pharmacotherapy for individuals and families. The next section reemphasizes the value of considering pharmacotherapy as a psychotherapeutic intervention, and the concluding section discusses combined treatment in the era of managed care.

■ OBSESSIVE-COMPULSIVE DISORDER AND THE "WORRY CIRCUIT"

The mind requires the brain in order to function. Therefore, abnormalities in brain function should correlate with abnormal mental functioning. These abnormalities in brain function should disappear with successful mind treatment.

However, we are in the middle of a profound paradigm shift. Most clinicians reflexively consider brain treatments to be medications (or electroconvulsive therapy), whereas psychotherapy is considered a mind treatment. However, psychotherapy treats the mind by altering the brain. Changes in the mind take place through changes in the brain.

This logic now boasts substantive research proof based on positron-emission tomography scans of the living brains of patients with obsessive-compulsive disorder treated with either medication (clomipramine) or behavior therapy (exposure and response prevention). Several areas of the brain appear to be hyperactive (hypermetabolic) in patients with obsessive-compulsive disorder. These areas include the orbital cortex of the frontal lobe and the caudate nucleus of the basal ganglia. Treatment success with either medications or behavior therapy shows close correlations between reductions in the standard measure of obsessive-compulsive disorder (Yale-Brown Obsessive Compulsive Scale; Goodman et al. 1989) and reductions in the hypermetabolic activity of the orbital cortex and the caudate nucleus. In other words, both medications and behavior therapy were effective in modulating brain function and correlated with a reduction in the symptoms of obsessive-compulsive disorder (Schwartz 1994).

The "worry circuit," which may be composed of the thalamus and cingulate gyrus as well as the caudate nucleus and orbital cortex (Baxter 1995), could also play a part in other obsessional disorders, including the ruminations of patients with depression and the worries of those with generalized anxiety disorder. Patients treated with selective serotonin reuptake inhibitors (SSRIs) report that their worries are still present but are not so intense; perhaps the medications reduce the firing rates of the circuit (L. R. Baxter, personal communication, February 1995).

One patient, for example, in the midst of marital turmoil, custody battles with her former husband, and high anxiety at work, raised her dose of paroxetine (Paxil) from 20 mg to 60 mg. When asked what the medication did, she replied: "It gives me a 'so what.'" Just as cognitive therapists encourage their patients to distance themselves from disturbing thoughts through challenging their beliefs with a "so what," SSRIs may help them accomplish the same end. The difference, of course, is that when the medication is withdrawn, the "so what" tends to disappear. On the other hand, can therapists think of medications like this as catalysts to reach states of mind that could be achievable by nonpharmacological means?

■ PSYCHOPHARMACOLOGY DURING THE STAGES OF PSYCHOTHERAPY

The tendency to dichotomize mind and brain, as suggested by René Descartes, has fostered the conceptual separation of pharmacotherapy and psychotherapy. Different clinicians sometimes perform different tasks as dictated by law, one giving pills, the other providing psychotherapy. Psychiatrists, who may perform both pharmacotherapy and psychotherapy, also tend to dichotomize the treatments within the clinical consultation, asking patients, "How are you doing with your medication?" In many instances, this encapsulated discussion serves the purpose of symptom-focused monitoring. There are times, however, when the alert psychotherapist can use the idea that medications may function as another psychotherapeutic intervention. To do so requires that psychotherapy be defined in generic terms rather than psychodynamic, cognitive, behavioral, systems, or existential-humanistic terms. The common-factors approach to psychotherapy integration offers this possibility (Norcross and Goldfried 1992).

Psychotherapy is based on an interpersonal relationship, following a problem-solving sequence that contains stages, each of which has discernible objectives. In the most common dyadic form, the pair must engage in a working alliance, define patterns to change, initiate and maintain change, and then terminate (Beitman 1987). Pharmacotherapy can aid as well as impede the accomplishment of the goals of each of these stages (Table 9–1).

Clinicians generally recognize that medications can aid in the engagement process and, conversely, that sometimes a strong working alliance must be developed in psychotherapy before patients will accept medications (Beitman 1991). Less well accepted are the psychodynamic and systems aspects of pharmacotherapy. The clinician who is willing to consider mind-brain crossings by speculating about the meaning of certain idiosyncratic patient reactions will be rewarded with a quicker, clearer definition of problematic psychological patterns. In addition, medications sometimes act as deviators from current family system equilibria, thereby creating disequilibria that may aid or subvert the therapeutic process. These modest conceptual shifts appear likely to aid in treatment efficiency, although research supporting these claims will be difficult to produce.

■ PHARMACOTHERAPY HIGHLIGHTS KEY DYSFUNCTIONAL PATTERNS

Medication Compliance and a Key Cognitive Pattern

Taking pills has meaning, and so does discontinuing them. Examining the reasoning behind irrational medication discontinuation and its consequences can serve as an illustration of a key dysfunctional pattern, as can any out-of-the-ordinary set of nonpharmacological behaviors. Consider the following examples.

TABLE 9–1. Stages of individual psychotherapy: a medication emphasis

Stage	Goals	Techniques	Content	Resistance	Transference	Countertransference
Engagement	Trust Credibility Alliance between self and observer	Convey empathic understanding Make effective suggestions Prescribe effective medications	Medication-responsive diagnosis	Are excessive side effects resistant to treatment?	For example, physician seen as malevolent or all-powerful	For example, physician failure to prescribe appropriately
Pattern search	Define problem patterns that, if changed, would lead to a desirable outcome	Questionnaires Homework Idiosyncratic meanings ascribed to medication	Does response to medication reflect a problem pattern?	Does pattern of nonadherence to medication regimen reflect a problem pattern?	Is key interpersonal pattern reflected in transaction about medication?	Medication prescription reflects distorted response to patient

TABLE 9–1. **Stages of individual psychotherapy: a medication emphasis** *(continued)*

Stage	Goals	Techniques	Content	Resistance	Transference	Countertransference
Change	Relinquish old pattern(s) Initiate new pattern(s) Practice new pattern(s)	Interpretation Cognitive change Behavioral suggestion Medication-induced change	Medication effects or insight about medication use accelerates change	Do new side effects suggest resistance to change?	Unresolved distortions may be signaled by a new medication issue inhibiting change	Sudden change in regimen reflects an attempt to undermine change

Source. Adapted from Beitman 1991.

Case 1

Mr. K, a 37-year-old travel agent, was being successfully treated for panic attacks with imipramine. He felt so normal that on a return trip from Hawaii he decided to discontinue the medication. On the plane, he had another panic attack. He reasoned that his panic attack was probably triggered by his fear of airplanes and his reluctance to return to the chaos of his family home. He seemed to ignore, however, that stopping his imipramine may have also contributed to the attack.

When asked whether he also had major blind spots in other parts of his life, he replied, "Yes, most definitely. My wife repeatedly points out to me the obvious things I miss with the children, and especially her." He was now open to new perspectives.

As-Needed Ingestion Illustrates a Key Interpersonal Pattern

Cognitive and behavioral therapists have long emphasized the great value of diaries in targeting symptomatic behavior. Patients can, in this way, use the many hours of the week not spent in therapy to gather data about their own difficulties. Patterns become more quickly recognized. One of the clear oversights of most dynamic therapies is the failure to use this simple, effective idea. As-needed ingestion of medications can be considered an example of dysfunctional behavior, just as panic attacks and increases in depression, smoking, and drinking serve as targets for psychotherapeutic efforts, as illustrated in the following case.

Case 2

Ms. L, a 55-year-old divorced insurance executive, had been taking butalbital (Fiortal) for many years, as prescribed by her family physician for headaches. Her psychiatrist asked her to record the times she took the medication. Much to her surprise, she discovered that she often took it shortly after being criticized or frustrated by a colleague or employer. This relationship helped to reduce her butalbital intake and facilitated her examination of this extreme sensitivity to frustration and criticism.

Transference and Countertransference

Like any other psychotherapeutic intervention, the transaction involving medications can involve significant distortions on the part of therapist and patient. Following are some brief descriptions.

Case 3

A 28-year-old male therapist had a 23-year-old female patient who had developed a strong sexualized transference to him. The therapist could not consider himself attractive to women because sexuality disturbed him. He offered the patient benzodiazepine. He was correct that someone was anxious, but he had selected the wrong person (Langs 1973).

Other examples include the following:

- Countertransference: A therapist is unconsciously angry at a patient, prescribes a side effect–prone medication, and tells the patient to come back in 3 months.
- Transference: A patient makes a suicide attempt with the therapist's medications, implying "you are killing me."
- Transference-countertransference: A patient tests the psychiatrist's degree of caring by demanding large doses of potentially addictive medications.
- Transference: As an indirect expression of anger at the therapist, a patient complains of excessive side effects from a medication previously taken for several months with no side effects.

Benzodiazepine Disinhibition Reveals Dysfunctional Patterns

In a small percentage of patients, benzodiazepines can unleash angry, aggressive, or paranoid states. A subset of these responses can highlight dysfunctional patterns, as illustrated in the following two cases.

Case 4

Ms. M, who was age 30, married, and unhappy and had been diagnosed with borderline personality disorder, took an overdose of alprazolam (Xanax) to forget everything. She was in therapy for 2 years and had begun to develop a strong attachment to her male psychiatrist but had up to this point behaved in a meek, passive, and compliant manner. On the overdose of alprazolam, she became an angry, vindictive, foul-mouthed adolescent. She hated her therapist, and no one could tell her what to do. She wanted what she wanted and was going to get it. A brief hospitalization was required. After another year of therapy, this part of her emerged in the transference, becoming at times psychotic as she demanded the body and soul of her psychiatrist. She was again angry and vindictive when she did not get her way. She could only dimly comprehend the unrealistic nature of her demands. The disinhibition response had revealed the future evolution of the transference.

Case 5

Ms. N, age 44, took a small dose of clonazepam for her panic attacks and felt better. She took a little more and felt even better. A little more, and she was full of energy and needed little sleep. But then she began to suspect that people in school were mistreating her daughter and that perhaps she needed to purchase a gun to protect her. Then she remembered that she supported gun control legislation and began to question her motives. Her psychiatrist suggested that she immediately discontinue taking the clonazepam. Her delusion dissipated. Further inspection of these paranoid thoughts revealed a close connection to her own childhood in which she was abused physically and emotionally by a highly religious set of parents who were part of a culture that tolerated the mistreatment of girls. In protecting her daughter, she was trying to do what no one had done for her as a child. This revelation set the stage for her moving away from her mother, who lived down the street, and finally claiming a life of her own away from the abusive culture of her parents. The move correlated with a steady diminution of her agoraphobic symptoms.

■ PHARMACOTHERAPY ALTERS MARITAL AND FAMILY DYNAMICS

Marital and family systems function at sometimes fragile equilibria. The introduction of change through medications and psychotherapy can sometimes reverberate through such systems to new states, some of which are desirable and some not. Sometimes one member improves, only to reveal dysfunction in another. Some families have much trouble adjusting to normalization of a depressed or anxious member who had been dysfunctional for many years. Some marriages dissolve when the apparently dysfunctional member improves. The following cases illustrate how medications in systems seem to trigger anticipated and sometimes unanticipated changes.

Medication Helps to Save Family Integrity

Occasionally, medications do what people hope they will do: almost magically turn around a deteriorating situation. Rather than facing divorce and custody battles, sometimes families are saved.

Case 6

Ms. O could no longer tolerate her husband's (Mr. P's) irritability and agoraphobia. The children could not be around him without being yelled at or criticized. Mr. P could not travel beyond the limits of their small town. He had been agoraphobic before they were married but had never bothered to tell her. Now they had two young children, and she could never go with Mr. P to her family gatherings 60 miles away or on any other small outing. Desperately, she sought help, not for herself but for him, from a psychiatrist in another town, because there was none in their town. Because Mr. P could not travel outside of his town limits, the psychiatrist talked to him on the phone. Mr. P had panic attacks and depression in addition to agoraphobia. With some trepidation, the psychiatrist prescribed imipramine without seeing the patient and emphasized a behavioral approach to his agoraphobia: travel increasingly greater distances from town. Mr. P became less depressed and less irritable while taking the imipramine and, after 2 years of prodding by Ms. O, showed up in the psychiatrist's office 30 miles away. They had gone to the annual family picnic. Ms. O was delighted.

Medications as Markers for Marital Difficulties

Tracking how medications fit into interpersonal transactions may illustrate interpersonal problems, as suggested by the next example.

Case 7

Ms. R, age 26, requested psychotherapy and medication 1 year after having made a serious suicide attempt in which she had taken her husband's antidepressant and lithium. Since her hospitalization, she had been maintaining herself on her husband's medications because her previous therapist had refused to refer her for them. (This use of his medications suggested that she was angry at her husband and that she was also dependent on him because she had used the pills in a suicide attempt and continued to need him to supply them for her afterward.)

Ms. R very much wanted independence from her husband. However, she continued to believe that she needed lithium, although she did not have bipolar disorder. Her psychiatrist prescribed lithium in low doses, allowing her to have her own supply. This intervention appeared to provide a deviation in the marital interaction pattern, which became amplified. She became more self-reliant; her husband could not accommodate her increased independence, and they eventually divorced (Beitman 1988).

Request for Pharmacotherapy for Spouse Helps Highlight a Marital Pattern

The alert clinician seeks to define single instances of a pattern of potentially dysfunctional behavior. The arena for such behavior includes the relationship between the patient and the therapist and the boundaries of that relationship.

Case 8

Mr. S wanted help with his marriage again. He had seen two previous therapists for the same reason. He had terminated with his
second therapist so that Mr. S's wife could be seen by that therapist after the couple had been in brief couples therapy with him.
Mr. S acquiesced to his wife in many other ways. She was agoraphobic with panic attacks, so they traveled little, usually
stayed on the first floor of hotels, and traveled only by car, stopping frequently. One day he brought home his favorite freshly
baked pie—cherry. She ate it all with no complaint from him.
After several sessions, Mr. S asked his psychiatrist to see his
wife for a medication evaluation, even though she had another
psychiatrist. "After all," said Mr. S, "you are the best in town in
treating panic disorder." His psychiatrist refused. Mr. S pleaded.
"Remember your last therapist. Remember the cherry pie," said
the psychiatrist. "You could at least call her," said Mr. S. "No!"
said the psychiatrist.

   This "No!" seems to have served as a model for Mr. S's increasing ability to not give in to his wife's demands and requests.
He no longer responded to her every whim. They separated, then
divorced. Her agoraphobia became significantly less severe after
the divorce. The refused consultation for pharmacotherapeutic
management had helped her to a positive change in her symptoms (Beitman 1991).

■ CATALYSTS FOR CHANGE

The emphasis of managed care on efficient, effective, high-quality
treatment is forcing mental health care practitioners to dramatically
reevaluate what they are doing and how they think about what they
are doing. One crucial conceptual shift involves the self-defined
role as therapist. Greenson (1967) characterized transference interpretation as "the ultimate and decisive instrument" (p. 39), echoing
many years of psychoanalytic belief in the therapist's words as scal-
pels of change. This ringing affirmation of the therapist's power to
change patients resembles the belief of many pharmacotherapists
(as well as psychopharmacologically naive therapists) that medica-

tions change people. In both scenarios, the psychopharmacologist-psychoanalyst, surgeon-like, operates on the passive psyche of the patient.

This interpersonal treatment schema for both medications and interpretations is being altered in the era of managed care. Therapists cannot assume the great burden that is implied. Patients must be clearly held accountable for instituting changes. And the therapist-psychopharmacologist is becoming a catalyst, an enzyme, for change.

How can this idea, well accepted among psychotherapists, be substantiated for pharmacotherapy? In a reported study, patients entering a trial for treatment of panic disorder with placebo or a new benzodiazepine completed the Stages of Change questionnaire (Beitman et al. 1994). This 32-item scale measured patient readiness to change across a four-category continuum. The study found that readiness to change predicted outcome in both the placebo and active drug groups. Subjects whose answers reflected a greater readiness to change underwent more positive changes than did those who seemed less ready to change. Therefore, medications, like other psychotherapeutic interventions, are incorporated into patients' own commitment to change and are coupled with their other coping strategies to bring about desired change.

This shift in pharmacological and psychotherapeutic views about medications underlies the cases reported in this chapter. Medications are sometimes simply another psychotherapeutic intervention.

■ COMBINED TREATMENT IN THE ERA OF MANAGED CARE

The pressures of cost savings are driving psychiatrists away from the practice of psychotherapy. The old mental health clinic model of the psychotherapy triangle—a pharmacotherapist, a nonmedical psychotherapist, and a patient—appears to be gaining ascendancy under managed care. Older psychiatrists, trained and experienced in long-term psychotherapy, are bitterly confronting a rapidly changing payment system that eliminates them from doing what they have grown to love.

If psychiatrists are to continue to do psychotherapy, the most likely venue will be as dual treaters using both pharmacotherapy and psychotherapy. The key question for future research is this: Under what conditions is it more cost-effective to have one person providing both medications and psychotherapy? Managers, whether physicians themselves or administrators, will want answers to this question. Here is a preliminary set of hypotheses.

Patients with severe DSM-IV (American Psychiatric Association 1994) diagnoses are likely to be more efficiently treated by one person, because the interaction between medications and psychotherapy may be tighter. For example, a patient with moderate major depression may respond quickly and easily to an SSRI; the medication will make him or her more readily able to use psychotherapy, whether provided by a pharmacotherapist or a psychotherapist. On the other hand, a person with bipolar disorder may start feeling good or bad because of a mix of influences—biochemical and environmental. Teasing out the distinction, making modest adjustments in medications, and understanding the interactions among pharmacotherapy, endocrine function, and psychosocial influences would be more efficiently accomplished by one person who is knowledgeable in biological as well as psychosocial areas.

Nevertheless, if psychiatrists are to continue practicing psychotherapy, they must learn to do so better. Psychiatrists' time costs more than social workers' time. Therefore, psychiatrists must learn how to be that much more efficient at providing therapy as they are paid relative to nonmedical practitioners.

Finally, in pharmacologically stabilized patients, a medication check takes perhaps 5 minutes, including rewriting the prescription. If the time allotted is 20–30 minutes, there could be adequate time for brief therapy.

The practice of medicine is being severely challenged by revolutionary changes in the system through which physicians are paid. Psychiatry's identity as a profession lies on the interface between mind and brain. Our practice straddles and integrates the concepts of psyche and soma. Combining pharmacotherapy and psychotherapy lies at the heart of clinical psychiatry.

■ REFERENCES

American Psychiatric Association: Diagnostic and Statistical Manual of Mental Disorders, 4th Edition. Washington, DC, American Psychiatric Association, 1994

Baxter LR: Neuroimaging studies of human anxiety disorders: cutting paths of knowledge through the field of neurotic phenomena, in Psychopharmacology: The Fourth Generation of Progress. Edited by Bloom FE, Kupfer DJ. New York, Raven, 1995, pp 66–101

Beitman BD: The Structure of Individual Psychotherapy. New York, Guilford, 1987

Beitman BD: Combining pharmacotherapy and psychotherapy: process considerations, in *Psychobiology and Psychopharmacology* (Directions in Psychiatry Monographs Series, Vol 2). Edited by Flach F. New York, WW Norton, 1988, pp 71–92

Beitman BD: Medications during psychotherapy: case studies of the reciprocal relationship between psychotherapy process and medication use, in Integrating Pharmacotherapy and Psychotherapy. Edited by Beitman BD, Klerman GL. Washington, DC, American Psychiatric Association, 1991, pp 21–43

Beitman BD, Beck NC, Deuser WE, et al: Patient stage of change predicts outcome in a panic disorder medication trial. Anxiety 1:64–69, 1994

Freud S: Project for a scientific psychology (1895), in The Standard Edition of the Complete Psychological Works of Sigmund Freud, Vol 1. Translated and edited by Strachey J. London, Hogarth Press, 1966, pp 281–397

Freud S: An outline of psychoanalysis (1940), in The Standard Edition of the Complete Psychological Works of Sigmund Freud, Vol 23. Translated and edited by Strachey J. London, Hogarth Press, 1964, pp 141–208

Goodman WK, Price LH, Rassmussen SA, et al: The Yale-Brown Obsessive-Compulsive Scale, II: validity. Arch Gen Psychiatry 46:1012–1016, 1989

Greenson RR: The Technique and Practice of Psychoanalysis, Vol 1. New York, International Universities Press, 1967

Langs R: Psychoanalytic Psychotherapy. Northvale, NJ, Jason Aronson, 1973

Norcross JC, Goldfried MR: Handbook of Psychotherapy Integration. New York, Basic Books, 1992

Schwartz JM: Cognitive-behavioral self-treatment for obsessive-compulsive disorder systematically alters cerebral metabolism: a mind-brain interaction paradigm for psychotherapists, in Obsessive-Compulsive Disorder: Diagnosis, Etiology, Treatment. Edited by Hollander E, Stein DJ. New York, Marcel Dekker, 1994, pp 88–122

Sperry L: Psychopharmacology and Psychotherapy. New York, Brunner/Mazel, 1995

INDEX

*Page numbers printed in **boldface** type refer to tables or figures.*